HALLUCINATIONS IN CLINICAL PSYCHIATRY

BRUNNER/MAZEL CLINICAL PSYCHIATRY SERIES
Series Editor: John G. Howells, M.D., F.R.C.Psych., D.P.M.

This Series aims to provide the clinician with information from the developing areas of psychiatry. Each volume in the Series constitutes a ready update of its subject by an acknowledged authority with the purpose of enhancing clinical practice.

BRUNNER/MAZEL CLINICAL PSYCHIATRY SERIES NO. 2

HALLUCINATIONS IN CLINICAL PSYCHIATRY =

A Guide for Mental Health Professionals

GHAZI ASAAD, M.D.

Clinical Associate Professor of Psychiatry
New York Medical College, Valhalla, New York

Director of Inpatient Psychiatric Services
Danbury Hospital, Danbury, Connecticut

BRUNNER/MAZEL, *Publishers* · NEW YORK

Library of Congress Cataloging-in-Publication Data
Asaad, Ghazi.
    Hallucinations in clinical psychiatry : a guide for mental health
professionals / Ghazi Asaad.
        p.   cm.—(Brunner/Mazel clinical psychiatry series ; no. 2)
    Includes bibliographical references.
    Includes index.
    ISBN 0-87630-592-3
    1. Hallucinations and illusions.   I. Title.   II. Series.
    [DNLM: 1. Hallucinations—diagnosis.   2. Hallucinations—therapy.
W1 BR917C no. 2 / WM 204 A798h]
RC553.H3A83 1990
616.89—dc20
DNLM/DLC
for Library of Congress   90-2125
                                                                     CIP

Published by
BRUNNER/MAZEL, INC.
19 Union Square
New York, New York 10003

Manufactured in the United States of America

10   9   8   7   6   5   4   3   2   1

Dedicated to my family with love.

Contents ⎯⎯

Introduction ═══

" 'We are going to get you, don't try to hide. We have to punish you for all the sins that you have committed.' That's what they are saying, can't you hear them? The voices are coming through the window," shouted Mr. K. "They are going to kill me. They will be waiting for me outside. You have to do something," he continued.

Mr. K. was a patient of mine 10 years ago in the beginning of my residency training in psychiatry. I was particularly struck by his intense and vivid hallucinatory symptoms, and by the degree of his conviction of their existence in reality. This experience stimulated my interest in hallucinations, and motivated me to explore these fascinating phenomena in order to learn more about their etiology and clinical significance. I went to the literature searching for answers, but I was rather disappointed to find that there was very little written about this important subject. Except for a few clinical reports, the majority of what I came across was concerned mainly with theoretical issues that could offer very little to the clinician who is working with patients with diverse clinical conditions and a wide variety of hallucinatory symptoms. My review of the literature and my extensive work with psychiatric patients resulted in the publication of my first paper on hallucinations (Asaad & Shapiro, 1986), which drew a significant amount of attention from mental health professionals, and prompted the invitation by Dr. John Howells, who presented the idea of writing a small book on hallucinations with particular orientation toward clinical matters. I was very excited about the idea and I went to work immediately. The project took over two years to complete, during which time I tried to gather all relevant information in the old and recent literature in order to provide the reader with a comprehensive overview of hallucinatory phenomena.

I offer this book as a clinical guide to assist the clinician in making a comprehensive clinical evaluation of hallucinatory symptoms as they present in various conditions, psychiatric and otherwise. Except for a few chapters that deal with theoretical background on the subject, the focus of most of this book is on clinical manifestations, diagnostic issues, and treatment approaches with regard to hallucinatory symptoms.

I have attempted in the final chapter to present a comprehensive theory that integrates psychodynamic, physiological, and neurochemical theories, and that provides an overall mechanism that can account for most hallucinatory phenomena. I hope that this contribution to the psychiatric literature will be of help to clinicians and interested readers.

Finally, I would like to acknowledge Bruce Shapiro, M.D., who contributed to the original paper (Asaad & Shapiro, 1986), which prompted the initiation of this academic adventure. Also, I would like to acknowledge Mark Ligorski, M.D., for his excellent editorial remarks, and Anne Marie Scozzafava for her immense secretarial support.

GHAZI ASAAD, M.D.

HALLUCINATIONS IN CLINICAL PSYCHIATRY ═

1

History of Hallucinations

Hallucinatory phenomena have been associated with insanity throughout history, and they have contributed a great deal to the mystery of "madness." In prehistoric times, mental illness was thought to be influenced by supernatural phenomena, especially the influence of spirits and demons. It is believed that trepanation of skulls performed in primitive cultures was meant as an attempt to liberate the afflicted patient from the evil spirits inside the head. Following that era, and as various civilizations started to rise around the world, attempts were made to understand the mysteries of mental illness. Far Eastern and Middle Eastern cultures viewed mental disorders within philosophical and religious concepts, giving mental disease an accepted and legitimate status. Greek and Roman cultures were dominated by literary, philosophical, and medical views that enhanced the understanding of mental illness. The medical concept of madness as elaborated in the Hippocratic writings (4th Century B.C.) centered on the interaction of the four bodily humors: blood, black bile, yellow bile, and phlegm. During the Greco-Roman period, there was greater acceptance of emotional manifestations of personality. This was particularly evident in dramatic productions, as seen in the plays of Euripides (ca. 484–407 B.C.) which demonstrate what might be described as an aesthetic appreciation of behavioral expressions of madness, such as hallucinations. These expressions were deliberately exaggerated for dramatic effect in several characters from his plays (Mora, 1985).

Plato (428–348 B.C.) believed that sickness of the psyche was due to discord among one's various personal traits or to ignorance of one's self and self deception. He described four types of madness: prophetic, ritual, poetic and erotic (Mora, 1985). Plato (1952) recognized the similarity between the dreams of sanity and the hallucinations of madness. He attempted to understand hallucinations and dreams through physiologic mechanisms and anatomic loci. He thought that rational thoughts along with perceptions occurred in the head, but that the part of the soul concerned with hallucinatory imagery and dreams was localized in the liver. Here it appears that Plato viewed hallucinations and perceptions as fundamentally different phenomena. He also maintained that the structures mediating dreams and hallucina-

1

tions were different from those underlying the perceptions of the waking state (Evarts, 1962).

Aristotle (384–322 B.C.) approached the various manifestations of human behavior from an empirical viewpoint that is more in line with current psychological understanding of behavior and mental illness. He believed that mysteries of madness represented ritual happenings that would eventually help in the healing process of mental disorder (Mora, 1985). Aristotle (1941) devoted a considerable amount of attention to dreams and hallucinations. Like Plato, he stressed the similarities between the two phenomena, but he differed from Plato in that he believed that the heart was the major organ of mind. Furthermore, he felt that dreams and waking perceptions were mediated by the same sensory mechanisms (Evarts, 1962).

During the Middle Ages (from the 4th to the 16th centuries), belief in the traditional concepts of the four bodily humors and of the influence of spirits on human behavior continued to prevail. The general belief was that mental illness could be cured by supernatural forces and saints. Although that era was considered a period of obscurations and superstition, some attention was given to the notions of localized functions in the brain, and physical therapies were applied as well. The 13th Century witnessed some progress in the area of understanding human behavior and mental illness, however, this was followed by an era of superstition and belief in the phenomenon of witchcraft that became prevalent in the 14th and 15th Centuries. During that period several treatises were published that contributed to the spread of this belief. The authors of the famous treatise "Malleus Maleficarum" (the Witches' Hammer) elaborated on the idea that a person who became delusional or hallucinated was considered to be possessed of the devil and to be a witch. "Malleus Maleficarum" became widely used as the handbook for inquisition for at least 2 hundred years (Zilboorg, 1935). The 16th Century marked an era of renaissance characterized by the culmination of humanitarian attitude toward mental patients and psychological understanding of their illness. The trend continued in the 17th and 18th Centuries (Mora, 1985).

The 19th Century witnessed a sharp rise in recreational use of hallucinogenic doses of Hashish and other drugs in Europe. This forced the French medical community to bring the phenomena of hallucinations under sharp scrutiny (West, 1975). Philippe Pinel (1745–1826) made a major contribution to the investigation of mental illness in general. He attempted to analyze and categorize symptoms in a very simple manner, and with great clarity. He also implemented what was known as "moral treatment" of mental illness. Pinel's favorite pupil, Jean Etienne Esquirol (1772–1840), dominated the psychiatric movement in France in the first half of the 19th Century. His 1837 textbook Des Maladies Mentales (Esquirol, 1965) became a classic both because of its clarity and its inclusion of statistics in the presentation of clinical matters. Esquirol studied hallucinatory phenomena, and was able to distinguish between illusions and hallucinations with regard to the presence or absence of external stimulus. In fact, his description became the basis for the current definition of hallucinations. In the decade following Esquirol's death in 1840, Moreau de Tours (1804–1884) continued the work on the hallucinatory phenomena. He described the occurrence of hallucinations under a wide variety of conditions, including psychological and physical stress. He studied the hallucinatory experience arising from drugs such as Stramonium and hashish. Whereas Esquirol pointed out the significant relationship between the content of dreams and hallucinations, Moreau pointed out the basic similarities in the functions of dreams and delirium. He suggested that hashish-derived hallucinations and mental illness were virtually identical psychical states resulting from central excitation. Other writers who contributed to the understanding of hallucinatory phenomena during that era included Brierre de Boismont (1798–1881) who described several instances of hallucinations occurring in the course of intense concentration, or musing. He extensively documented the occurrence of hallucinatory symptoms in several mental disorders (West, 1975).

The second half of the 19th Century witnessed more advances in the area of mental disorders and hallucinations. Pierre Janet (1859–1947) described the occurrence of hallucinations during somnambulism and other dissociative reactions. Interest in hallucinations soon spread from France to other European countries such as Germany, Austria, and England, and several other people continued the work on illusions and hallucinations.

Before the turn of the Century, Hughlings Jackson (1834–1911) made a significant contribution to the theory of hallucinations. He was able to combine the philosophical speculation of the past with knowledge of cerebral function that was available at that time in order to formulate his concepts. Jackson stated that dreaming was physiologic insanity, and he used neurophysiological terms to explain cerebral processes. Jackson hypothesized that differences in strength of neuronal discharge were responsible for the variations in the intensity of ideation and perception. He suggested that the elimination of an inhibitory process during sleep and insanity leads to strong discharges that cause dreams and hallucinations (Evarts, 1962).

During the early part of the 20th Century, neurologists and psychiatrists continued to study hallucinatory phenomena during the first three decades, however, during the next 20 years there was an apparent decrease in interest in the subject. Sigmund Freud's (1856–1939) contribution to hallucinations was largely limited to his formulation that pointed out their similarities to dreams. He maintained that like dreams, hallucinations represent a breakthrough of preconscious or unconscious material into consciousness in the form of sensory images in response to psychological situations and needs. The Freudian era was largely dominated by interest in "neuroses" and psychoanalysis which may have contributed to the relative decline in interest in hallucinations and psychosis in general. However, during the early part of the second half of the 20th Century, interest in hallucinations was revived.

This was due, in large part, to the surge of work on hallucinogenic drugs. In addition, new approaches to experimental psychopathology such as sensory isolation, sensory overload, sleep deprivation, and the new understanding of the phenomenology of dreaming in sleep research provided a significant amount of data in support of several theories that attempted to explain the phenomena of hallucinations. These theories will be reviewed in Chapter 5.

According to Webster's Third International Dictionary, "hallucinate" was derived from the Latin word "hallucinatus" or "alucinatus" from the Greek origin, "hyalein" or "alyein," which means "to wonder in mind." The word was first used in the English language in the 16th Century in a translation of a tract by Lavater who used the word to refer to "ghosts and spirits walking by nyght" (Sarbin & Juhasz, 1975). Subsequently, the word was used to describe behavior that is intended as serious by the person, but is perceived as heedless or foolish by an observer. "Hallucination" became a technical term in psychology and medicine in the hands of Esquirol in the 19th Century, who described clearly the meaning of the term. His description laid the foundation for the current definition of hallucinations. Bleuler (1950) defined hallucinations as "perceptions without corresponding stimuli from without." Several other definitions may be encountered in the psychiatric literature. In the course of this book, hallucinations are defined as "perceptions that occur in the absence of corresponding external stimuli" (Asaad & Shapiro, 1986).

2 ═

Phenomenology of Hallucinations

Perception is the awareness of objects and relations in the surrounding environment in response to the stimulation of peripheral sense organs, as distinct from the awareness that results from memory. Any impairment in the perceptual apparatus may set the stage for delusions, hallucinations, illusions, and a variety of misinterpretations of reality (Linn, 1985).

Hallucinations are generally defined as perceptions that occur in the absence of corresponding external stimuli. Such perceptions may involve any of the senses. Consequently, several types of hallucinations may be experienced: auditory, visual, tactile, olfactory, and gustatory. Complex or mixed hallucinations also occur.

Auditory hallucinations are usually perceived as words or sentences heard by the patient as remarks or comments concerning him or her. The patient may experience two voices talking about him or her in the third person; they may debate in an approving or antagonistic manner, or they may command the patient to act in a certain way. The voices may be heard as coming from inside the head or from outside. This type of hallucination is frequently described in the course of schizophrenia, manic or depressive episodes with psychotic features, and other "functional" psychotic conditions. Similar hallucinations may occur less frequently in organic mental disorders, including psychotic conditions induced by pharmacologic agents or psychedelic substances. In such instances, auditory hallucinations are usually less formed, and may be perceived as music, or simple sounds such as whispers, ticking of a clock, footsteps, a closing door, and other indistinct noises. It is important to note here that simple auditory hallucinations are sometimes reported in schizophrenia and other "functional" psychotic states. Conversely, complex auditory hallucinations such as voices or sentences are also reported in organic psychoses (Asaad & Shapiro, 1986). The differential diagnosis of hallucinations is discussed in Chapter Sixteen.

Although auditory hallucinations are thought to be private events, some writers (Green & Preston, 1981) have reported that such hallucinations often are associated with movement of the laryngeal musculature. It has been suggested that the patient is uttering subvocally the same words he or she may be hearing in the hallucinations. The correlation between these subvocalizations and the mechanism of auditory hallucinations is still unclear.

Visual hallucinations are usually perceived as images of people, animals, or other objects depending on the patient's clinical condition. These images might take the form of an event occurring in front of the patient, or they may simply appear to the patient as pictures or symbols with certain meanings. They may also be less complex and manifest in simple objects such as stars, lines, circles, flashes of light, or colors. Visual hallucinations are mostly reported in organic mental disorders including reactions to drugs and psychedelic substances; however, they also occur in schizophrenia and other "functional" psychotic states.

Flashbacks are spontaneous recurrences of visual hallucinations and illusions that occur in some people who have a history of repeated ingestion of drugs. Such experiences occur during a drug-free period and resemble those hallucinations experienced during the active stage of drug administration. These flashbacks may occur several months after the last use of the drug (Horowitz, 1969). The exact cause of such phenomena is still unclear. Intrusive visual images of traumatic experiences have been reported to occur as flashbacks in patients with post-traumatic stress disorder (Brett & Ostroff, 1985).

Lilliputian hallucinations are visual hallucinations in which the patient experiences seeing people who appear greatly reduced in size. These hallucinations occur typically as a result of Atropine's, and other anticholinergic agents', toxicity. They may also occur in the other organic mental disorders as well as "functional" psychotic states.

Autoscopic phenomena (Lukianowicz, 1958) refer to hallucinatory experiences in which all or part of the person's own body is perceived as appearing in a mirror. The image is usually transparent and colorless. It appears suddenly and imitates the person's movements. Other types of hallucinations may be experienced concurrently. The person is usually aware of the unreality of the experience. This condition is rare and poorly understood, but is probably caused by diffuse organic cerebral pathology. It has been reported in migraine, epilepsy, delirium, and in a variety of other diffuse cerebral diseases. Occasionally it occurs in schizophrenia and depressive psychosis. It has been hypothesized that the phenomenon is due to a highly developed visual memory sense with strong eidetic imagery. Psychodynamic issues may also be involved (Lishman, 1987). For some, this experience may occur once in a lifetime, but for others it may happen repeatedly.

Tactile hallucinations (also known as *Haptic hallucinations*) are false perceptions of touch. These hallucinations may take the form of insects crawling on the skin. This condition is known as *formication*. Tactile hallucinations are generally experienced in organic conditions such as delirium tremens, cocaine and amphetamine intoxications, but they also occur in psychotic conditions such as schizophrenia.

Olfactory hallucinations are false perceptions of smell, whereas *gustatory hallucinations* are false perceptions of taste. These conditions are reported in temporal lobe epilepsy and uncinate gyrus fits. They also occur in some patients with psychiatric disorders such as schizophrenia.

As noted earlier, more complex or mixed types of hallucinations may be experienced by certain patients. Schizophrenics often experience *cenesthetic hallucinations* which are reported as altered states of body organs or peculiar visceral sensations that could not be perceived under appropriate physiological conditions due to the lack of receptor apparatus to explain the sensations, e.g., burning sensation in the brain or feeling of blood flow inside blood vessels. These hallucinations are rare and poorly understood (Asaad & Shapiro, 1986).

Patients under the influence of psychedelic drugs may experience *synesthetic hallucinations*. In this condition the patient perceives a colorful visual hallucination after hearing a loud noise, or may have auditory hallucinations in response to a bright light. This phenomenon probably occurs because of drug induced cortical hypersensitivity that allows a strong stimulus in one area to trigger other areas of the cortex (Asaad & Shapiro, 1986).

Kinesthetic hallucinations are perceptions of the movement of body parts that are not actually moving. Patients may perceive sensations or movements of body parts that have been amputated. The phantom limb syndrome is a good example of such hallucinations (Lishman, 1987).

Hypnagogic hallucinations are false sensory perceptions occurring during the period prior to falling asleep. *Hypnopompic hallucinations* are similar experiences that happen during the transition from sleep to wakefulness. These hallucinations may contain both auditory and visual elements of great clarity and intensity. Hypnagogic and hypnopompic hallucinations may be experienced by patients with narcolepsy and hysteria. However, they are also frequent in healthy individuals (West, 1975).

Hallucinosis is an organically based hallucinatory phenomenon in the absence of other psychotic symptoms. The patient is usually alert, oriented, and shows insight into the problem. Alcoholic hallucinosis is a good example of such hallucinations.

Negative hallucinations refer to the failure of a person to perceive a stimulus despite having a physiologically intact nervous system. Such a condition may occur as part of the syndrome of hysteria, or it can be induced through hypnosis.

Pseudohallucinations refer to conditions in which the person experiences the hallucinations under certain conditions, but is fully aware of the unreality of the experience. An example of such hallucination happens during grief periods when some people may hear the voice or see the image of the deceased person (Sedman, 1966).

Illusions are defined as false sensory perceptions of real external stimuli that may be misinterpreted and perceived in a distorted way. Like hallucinations, these perceptions may involve any of the senses, however, visual and auditory illusions are more frequent than other types (Asaad, 1989).

3

Hallucinations, Illusions, and Delusions

The perception of the external world around us is heavily dependent on the state of the nervous system starting with the peripheral sensory organs and ending with the cortex. It is also influenced by our past experiences, current anticipations, and the various environmental factors interacting during the experience (Segal, 1970). As indicated earlier, any impairment in the perceptual apparatus may set the stage for hallucinations, illusions, delusions, and other related phenomena depending on the nature of the impairment, as well as the influence of the environmental factors.

Illusions have been defined as false sensory perceptions of actual external sensory stimuli. These then become misinterpreted and perceived unrealistically with variable degrees of insight depending on the circumstances of the individual and the conditions under which the phenomena occur. Although, like hallucinations, these perceptions may involve any of the senses, visual and auditory illusions are more frequent than other types. Until Jean Etienne Esquirol (1772–1840) clarified the difference between the two phenomena, the terms hallucinations and illusions were being used interchangeably with confusion and inconsistent definitions. Esquirol emphasized the presence of an external source of stimulation in the case of illusions, as opposed to hallucinations. The original concept offered by Esquirol in his textbook *Des Maladies Mentales* (1837) laid the foundation for the current definitions of the two phenomena (Esquirol, 1965).

Illusions may occur in normal people under various circumstances. They can occur in clear or altered states of consciousness. When the individual is in a clear state of consciousness, the experience is generally simple and isolated. A frightened individual in a darkened surrounding may perceive a tree trunk nearby as someone who is ready to attack. More elaborate types of illusions may occur in certain toxic states in which clouding of consciousness may develop. Examples include alcohol withdrawal syndrome, known as delirium tremens. In such conditions, the simple images perceived may be elaborated into complex images with resultant fantasies. The patient may perceive cracks in the wall as snakes crawling, or perceive the sound of footsteps as someone banging on the door. Other symptoms may appear, such as hallucinations, delusions, and agitation (Feldman & Bender, 1970). Organic mental disorders, in general, predispose to such kinds of experiences. It is commonly known that people under the influence of psychedelic substances often report various types of illusions involving real objects that appear in altered shapes and colors. Alterations of time and space may also occur. A short distance may seem much longer than it is in reality, and a few minutes may feel like hours.

Illusions that occur in the course of organic mental disorders or under the influence of substances may be accompanied by pseudohallucinations or true hallucinations. Patients with visual disorders or partial blindness resulting from opacities of the ocular media such as cataract may have illusory vision. Illusions also occur in psychotic conditions. A schizophrenic patient may hear an insulting remark in the chime of a clock. Although such an experience may be referred to as an illusion, it actually borders on the hallucinatory side (Kaplan & Sadock, 1985).

Delusions are false beliefs firmly held by the patient and unlikely to be shaken by reasoning or logical explanation. Whereas illusions are considered a product of perceptual distortions, delusions represent ideational distortions. Ideas of reference represent a form of delusions that are based on ideational distortions of events or environmental cues. Here, the patient may interpret a casual look by a passerby as a signal for impending danger. Such ideas may become more elaborate and develop into true delusions. Delusions are actually generated in the patient's mind in the absence of any reality based events. Paranoid delusions and bizarre delusions are examples of such phenomena, and they are frequently reported in schizophrenia.

On a theoretical level, one can compare delusions which represent false beliefs that have no basis in reality with hallucinations which also represent false perceptions that have no basis in reality. The parallel here is very interesting, as it identifies two spheres of awareness, one that utilizes sensory perceptual pathways by which illusions and hallucinations are perceived, and another that utilizes cognitive ideational pathways, by which ideas of reference and delusions are experienced. Within each sphere, the degree of the distortion may vary, and usually depends on several psychodynamic, biological, and environmental factors. The spectrum of pathology in the sensory perceptual sphere may begin with mild distortion of sensory stimuli under certain conditions leading to illusionary experiences, and end with an extreme state of hallucinations and perceptions that have no basis in the external world. Along the spectrum, variable degrees of perceptual distortions and experiences may be encountered. Similarly, the spectrum of pathology in the cognitive ideational sphere may begin with mild distortions of certain remarks or events as in the case of ideas of reference, and end with severe form of delusional thinking that is totally out of touch with reality. Here, too, one can find variable degrees of ideational distortion and false beliefs along that spectrum.

The concept of the spectrum within the sensory perceptual sphere and the cognitive ideational sphere, along with the parallel drawn between the two spheres, raises the question of the relationship between hallucinations and delusions. Strauss (1969) suggested that "hallucinations and delusions represent points on dimensions of perceptual and ideational continua function, rather than two separate entities." The theory states that early in the disease process the patient experiences breakdown in the perceptual constancy which results in illusions and hallucinations. Later, and as the condition deteriorates, the patient develops breakdown in the ideational capacity leading to ideas of reference and delusions. Such a concept implies that having delusional thinking constitutes a more severe or advanced stage of psychopathology than having hallucinations. This notion is not supported by current clinical examples. Furthermore, both hallucinations and delusions are often experienced by the patient at the same time. This situation cannot be explained by the continuum theory proposed by Strauss.

It would seem more useful if the concept of the continuum is applied to each symptom separately wherein the degree of impairment of ego functions can be utilized in the assessment of the illness and may offer certain advantages to treatment modalities. Pseudohallucinations and hallucinations can be seen as points on a continuum with insight and reality testing being the reference guidelines. At an ideational level, one can see hypochondriacal fears and somatic delusions also as points on that continuum.

Zigler and Levine (1983) reviewed several reports that argued that hallucinations and delusions are closely related phenomena and may, in fact, represent adjacent segments on an underlying continuum. These segments can be mixed or overlapped in certain instances, leading to pathological phenomena labeled as "delusional perception" or "perceptual delusions." This may suggest that the sensory perceptual distortion is supported by a cognitive ideational component experienced simultaneously by the patient.

Approaching the same concept from a developmental point of view, Zigler and Levine (1983) suggested that schizophrenic patients who manifest delusions were found to be at a higher developmental level as assessed by a premorbid social competence index, than those who suffered hallucinations. The social competence of patients having both symptoms tended to fall between the two groups, although they may be viewed clinically as members of a "sicker" group than those patients suffering from either hallucinations or delusions, respectively. This observation led the authors to hypothesize that delusions represent a higher developmental phenomenon than do hallucinations. They added that this hypothesis is consistent with other views that consider hallucinations to be closely related to other developmentally immature phenomena, such as dreams, eidetic imagery, and imaginary playmates.

Hallucinations often occur with delusions during psychotic states. Both phenomena seem to complement each other and serve similar functions in expressing unconscious psychological conflicts. However, hallucinations offer concrete symbolic expression of the conflict that may be also expressed in more abstract forms through delusions. The predominance of hallucinatory symptoms in certain patients may reflect the cognitive limitations of those individuals, who may choose concrete ways to express stressful internal experiences. Others with higher cognitive abilities may resort to delusional forms to express the same experiences.

Within the hallucinatory phenomenon itself, the concept of the continuum could be applied with regard to imagery, pseudohallucinations, and hallucinations. Here, reality testing seems to be the critical factor that might move the experience on the continuum in one direction or another, depending on the degree of the impairment.

Imagery is defined as an experience appearing in inner subjective space and lacking the concrete reality of perception. Such experiences are usually self-evoked and under the control of the will (Sedman, 1966). Imagery experiences involve mostly visual and auditory perceptions that can be very clear and vivid. Furthermore, imagery tends to occur during stages of clear consciousness, and it varies from person to person. According to Sedman (1966), people with personality organizations associated with attention seeking and obsessive compulsive features seem to be capable of experiencing imagery more than others. In any event, imagery does not reflect any specific psychopathological state, and, in fact, it is considered to be part of normal experience. However, the content of the imagery may be determined by significant underlying psychodynamic factors.

Pseudohallucinations are defined as hallucinations that are experienced by the subject who, at the time of the experience, is fully aware of the unreality of the perceptions. The perceptions are usually in the visual or auditory modalities. However, olfactory and tactile sensations have been reported by many individuals. They may occur as single experiences in the individual's life, as in the case of grief reactions, or they may occur frequently under various circumstances. Such perceptions are usually clear with full sensory details. In the initial part of the experience, the person may not be able to make a critical judgment concerning the unreality of the perception, but in a few moments, that distinction becomes clear. Sedman (1966) found that pseudohallucinations reported during states of clear consciousness tend to occur more frequently in females and in people with premorbid personality exhibiting self-insecurity and attention seeking traits. He also found a high incidence of sexual frigidity in those female patients. On the other hand, Sedman (1966) noted that when pseudohallucinations occurred during half-waking states, such sex difference and personality profile did not seem to apply. Hypnagogic and hypnopompic hallucinations are good examples of pseudohallucinations during half-waking periods, and they do not carry any specific pathological significance. Pseudohallucinations are rarely reported during states of clouding of consciousness, such as deliria states. The relationship between pseudohallucinations and hysteria will be addressed in Chapter Fourteen.

True hallucinations are experienced and accepted by the patient as real perceptions. It is obvious that reality testing must be impaired in order for this symptom to appear. True hallucinations usually occur in a setting of clear consciousness as in schizophrenia and other "functional" psychotic states. In such conditions, auditory hallucinations constitute the predominant form, although other types may predominate in certain patients. True hallucinations may also occur in a setting of clouded consciousness in patients with organic mental disorders—delirious states—where visual hallucinations are experienced more frequently. True hallucinations are rarely reported during half-waking states.

Although the continuum concept moving from imagery to pseudohallucinations to hallucinations is an interesting one, the complexity of the hallucinatory phenomena and the variety of disorders and states that present with such symptomatology lead to the conclusion that several other factors have to be involved in the process. Therefore, the simple continuum model may only be partially relevant and useful in order to understand the phenomenological aspects of hallucinations (Asaad, 1989).

SUMMARY

Illusions are related to hallucinations in the sense that both phenomena involve perceptual disturbances of various sensory organs. However, the two phenomena differ in a fundamental way: external stimulus is present in illusions, but not in hallucinations.

Hallucinations and delusions are similar in that both states reflect significant impairment in reality testing, which allows the individual to experience sensations or ideas that have no basis in reality. The two phenomena are different, however, in that hallucinations utilize perceptual pathways, whereas delusions utilize ideational pathways.

Imagery, pseudohallucinations, and hallucinations seem to lie on a perceptual continuum that is influenced by changes in reality testing that may move the experience in one direction or another. Similarly, ideas of reference and delusions can be seen along an ideational continuum that is also influenced by changes in reality testing.

Hallucinations, illusions, and delusions are psychiatric symptoms that can occur simultaneously or independently, as determined by the underlying pathology.

4 ═══

Hallucinations, Dreams, and REM Sleep

In his original work on dreams, Freud (1953) felt that hallucinations were very similar to dreams. In fact, he attempted to establish the relations between dreams and mental diseases. Freud felt that dreams represent psychotic states, or at least have great resemblance to psychosis. In this process, thoughts are transformed into images, mainly of a visual sort, that is, word presentations are taken back to corresponding "thing" presentations. According to Jones (1962), Freud pointed out that there was a major difference between dreams and hallucinations, where hallucinations cannot be explained by a simple regression of the same kind that takes place in dreams. He concluded that in the case of hallucinations, something has to happen to the "criteria of reality" as well. Thus, according to Freud, hallucinations can never be an early symptom of psychosis, but come about only if there is already a major impairment of the ego. However, clinical evidence indicates that in some cases hallucinations can in fact precede other psychotic symptoms. This observation raises some questions about Freud's original conceptualization of hallucinations.

Freud felt that dreams utilize predominantly visual images, and to a lesser extent, auditory images. Impressions belonging to other senses may occasionally be involved. He noted that thoughts and ideas do occur in dreams in the form of residues of verbal presentations, the content of which behaves like images that are closer to perceptions than they are to memory related presentations. Thus, dreams replace thoughts by hallucinations. An example that illustrates this concept is that of a person who falls asleep with the memory of a series of musical notes in mind; the memory becomes transformed into a hallucination of the same melody. Within this conceptualization, no distinction is made between visual and acoustic presentations (Freud, 1953).

Another link between hallucinations and dreams was referred to by Freud when he indicated that both hallucinations and dreams serve as a regressive experience for wish fulfillment. The unconscious wishful impulses are played out readily during dreams when most mature defenses are lifted through the

14

relaxation of the censorship mechanism. A similar process takes place in hallucinations where unconscious wishful impulses try to make themselves effective in daytime as well.

The indisputable analogy between dreams and hallucinations outlined by Freud presented a great challenge to the theory of dream life. Until that time, the prevailing perspective regarded dreaming as a useless and disturbing process, and as the expression of a reduced activity of the mind.

Psychotic states, whether in schizophrenia or in drug-induced psychosis, share with dreams the loss of ego boundaries. This seems to allow hallucinatory experience to emerge freely to fulfill certain wishes or express unconscious conflicts.

The regressive loss of reality testing and ego boundaries leads to a chaotic condition with loss of temporal continuity. It has been indicated that in dreams and psychoses there is a complete lack of sense of time. This is observed in some schizophrenic patients and in people who are under the influence of hallucinogenic drugs who report feeling "timelessness," time "standing still," or time "slowed down."

Fischman (1983) concluded that there is a fundamental process common to dreams, hallucinogenic drug states, and acute psychoses. This process involves sustained "disruption of the ego's ongoing synthesis of the various self-representations into a continuous, coherent self." The process is closely related to the loss of reality testing and the emergence of primary process seen in all three conditions. Furthermore, it appears that in all of these states there is a tendency toward concretization, with loss of abstract thinking.

Before Freud, Aristotle (1941) proposed that the hallucinations of madness resulted from aberrant functioning of those mechanisms that normally produce hallucinations during sleep in the form of dreaming. In recent years, the discovery of REM sleep and its relationship to dreaming has offered some clues to the relationship between the two phenomena. Feinberg (1970) reported that there is much more mental activity during sleep than was previously suspected. People awakened during REM sleep report mental activity characterized by visual imagery of a bizarre and implausible nature, associated with affective involvement of the dreamer. On the other hand, awakening from non-REM sleep is less likely to be accompanied by such mental activities. This essential distinction between REM sleep and non-REM sleep periods concerning the mental activities reported by individuals has led to the assumption that the mechanism responsible for hallucinations is closely related to the mechanism of dreaming during REM sleep. However, it is important to mention here that in a small but definite number of instances, very typical dream reports are elicited from people awakening from non-REM sleep (Feinberg, 1970).

The amounts of REM sleep recorded in hallucinating schizophrenic patients did not differ significantly from those of the nonhallucinating patients. However, the results of sleep studies in delirium were more positive. Here, high levels of REM sleep were observed and, in some instances, this was associated with hallucinations (Feinberg, 1970).

Itil (1970) noted that electroencephalographical recordings during dreaming states show patterns similar to those produced by certain hallucinogens. Hallucinations, experimentally induced by anticholinergic and indole hallucinogens, have been correlated with a decrease of alpha waves and an increase of high-frequency, fast activity in the EEG. LSD (an indole hallucinogen) induced accleration and flattening of EEG activity during the hallucinatory experience reported by the subject, whereas Ditran and Atropine (anticholinergic hallucinogens) induced both very slow and very fast activity during the confusional delirious state experienced by the subject. Computerized analysis of the EEG pattern during REM sleep dreaming states has shown an increase in both slow and fast activities as compared to the activities recorded during the waking and drowsiness states. These findings have supported the hypothesis suggesting similar neurophysiological mechanism for hallucinations and dreams.

Further evidence in support of the theory that emphasizes the presence of some relationship between hallucinations and REM sleep was presented by Dement et al. (1969), who proposed that "a defective serotonin gating mechanism allowed some phasic events of REM sleep to intrude into the waking state." The hypothesis states that Pontine-geniculate-occipital (PGO) waves, normally confined to REM sleep, may emerge into the non-REM waking states. Hallucinatory-like behavior that coincided with the emergence of PGO waves during waking states was observed in animals. It was proposed that PGO waves were the "minimal neural substrate" of dream images, and that the hallucinations of schizophrenia may be produced by a similar mechanism. This theory was later challenged by several researchers (Fischman, 1983).

Fischer (1969) suggested that a common denominator of drug-induced hallucinations and of REM dreaming states is the raised level of arousal. This level of arousal is characterized by a high sensory to motor ratio causing disequilibrium between the internal and the external sensory awareness and decreased motor responsiveness.

At a biochemical level, Fischman (1983) summarized the biological considerations involved in REM sleep, non-REM sleep, and hallucinations. He reported the experimental work of others that showed that the serotonergic outflow from the dorsal raphe nucleus decreases progressively as the animal transitions from the waking state through non-REM sleep and then into REM sleep. He added that these serotonergic neurons become virtually silent during REM sleep. Fischman also noted that norepinephrine-containing neurons of the locus ceruleus follow a similar pattern of activity, but to a lesser extent. It is important to mention here that central serotonergic levels have been shown to be reduced in cases of hallucinations induced by a number of hallucinogenic drugs such as Lysergide (LSD), Mescaline, and Amphetamine (Asaad & Shapiro, 1986).

Thus, the phenomenological similarity of dreams (which occur most vividly in REM sleep) and drug-induced hallucinations might be mediated, at least in part, by the inactivation of central serotonergic neurotransmission. Furthermore, it is believed that serotonin has a role in the direct inhibition of dopaminergic neurotransmission in the substantia nigra, neostriatum, and nucleus accumbens. Decreased central serotonin level will remove the inhibitory effects leading to increased dopaminergic activity which may contribute to the emergence of hallucinatory symptoms during hallucinogenic drug states and the emergence of dreams during REM sleep (Fischman, 1983).

Prolonged periods of sleep deprivation sometimes lead to hallucinations and other psychotic symptoms (Mullaney et al., 1983). Additionally, it is well known that recovery sleep following long sleep deprivation is usually characterized by significant increase in REM sleep. The exact correlation between hallucinatory experiences during sleep deprivation and the increase in REM sleep during the recovery phase is unclear.

Further evidence that links hallucinations to REM sleep states was noted by Snyder (1983). He reported that some passengers experienced visual and auditory hallucinations accompanied by sleep paralysis after waking up from several hours of sleep during a 13-hour flight. He concluded that rapid time zone shift ("jet lag" syndrome) could have specific effects on sleep cycle, leading to altered REM onset, length, and periodicity.

Hypnagogic (sleep-inducing) and hypnopompic (sleep terminating) hallucinations are closely related to dreams. Savage (1975) considered these hallucinations to fall between dreams and actual hallucinations. He suggested that hypnagogic hallucinations sometimes become incorporated into dreams. Similarly, he felt that dreams could turn into hypnopompic hallucinations.

SUMMARY

Clinical, physiological, and biochemical evidence has been presented in support of the hypotheses correlating hallucinations, dreams, and REM sleep. Despite the similarities outlined above between hallucinations and dreams, the two phenomena are far from being identical. Dreams are accepted as normal physiological phenomena, whereas hallucinations generally represent an underlying pathological process except for some states mentioned later in this book. Furthermore, the hallucinatory phenomena are too complex and variable to be explained simply by the physiological process of REM sleep and dreams.

5 =

Etiology and Psychopathology

Hallucinations are viewed as major symptoms of psychiatric disorders and certain medical conditions that are associated with psychoses. Despite all the advances in research in the field of mental illness, no single mechanism has been shown to account for the etiology or pathogenesis of hallucinatory phenomena. On the other hand, there is a substantial body of knowledge that points toward multiple etiological factors that seem to contribute to the formation and manifestation of hallucinations. These factors include psychodynamic, psychophysiological, and neurochemical components.

PSYCHODYNAMIC THEORIES

Since the times of Plato (428–348 B.C.) and Aristotle (384–322 B.C.), hallucinations and dreams have been viewed as similar phenomena. More recently, Freud pointed out the similarities and differences emphasizing that both phenomena represent a breakthrough of preconscious or unconscious material into consciousness in response to certain psychological situations or needs. He felt that in hallucinations words and thoughts are transformed into sensory material that gets projected and then consciously experienced as coming from the external world. Such experiences, although they may lack a basis in reality, are nevertheless perceived as real by the patient who is usually convinced that they are caused by external stimuli. Furthermore, these experiences may, in fact, constitute an actual part of the patient's mental life.

Within the psychoanalytic theory, hallucinations are considered to represent projections of inner conflicts during psychotic states when the ego is weakened and most mature defense mechanisms prove unsuccessful. The projected psychological material may be expressed through any of the senses, depending on the nature of the conflict and its symbolic significance. In all cases, the contents of the hallucinations generally reflect the underlying psychodynamic situations and needs, such as fulfillment of a repressed wish, enhancement of self-esteem, feeling of guilt, satisfaction of repressed impulses, or desire for a more satisfying reality.

Feeling of guilt is best expressed in spoken language. Patients with such

18

an underlying psychodynamic may report hearing voices telling them that they are bad and worthless. In this context, accusatory voices may represent the projected superego critical voice.

Feinberg (1962) proposed that the hallucinations may, at times, involve an ego rather than a superego function. Within this concept, he theorized that traumatic events that lead to the development of schizophrenia may take place at a critical period in development when language mastery is still in progress. According to Feinberg, this disturbance in language development will then contribute to hallucinations of schizophrenia. Arieti (1974) proposed that schizophrenic patients hear hallucinatory voices only when they expect to hear them. Arieti explained that patients put themselves into a "listening attitude," wherein they believe that the voices will talk, and soon after they begin to hear the voices.

Fears of some aspects of the personality, such as aggressive elements, are well symbolized by visual hallucinations. In such instances, the patient may project his or her hostile and aggressive wishes to the external world, and then experience them as coming from the outside in the form of visual hallucinations consisting of the sight of terrifying animals.

Similarly, other sensory modalities may be chosen based on their ability to symbolize the particular material seeking expression. For example, a patient who has poor self-esteem and sees herself as a rotten person may then develop, during a psychotic state, the olfactory hallucination that a bad odor emanates from her body. Another patient who feels that his wife is trying to kill him may develop a gustatory hallucination in which he experiences a particular taste in his mouth because he believes that his wife has poisoned his food. A manic patient who is sexually preoccupied and aroused may report a tactile hallucination in which he feels that someone is touching his genital organs.

It is generally accepted that during psychotic states the ego boundaries lose their cathexis leading to major impairment of reality testing where internal processes can no longer be distinguished from external ones (Fischman, 1983). With this, secondary process becomes impaired, allowing the primary process to predominate. Freud indicated that the primary process transformation that occurs in dreams involves the transformation of thoughts into images. The same mechanism seems to apply in the case of hallucinations in which thoughts and concepts are transformed into sounds, images, or other forms of perceptions. More recently, Arieti (1974) introduced the term "perceptualization of the concept," to refer to the mental process that takes place in the evolution of schizophrenic hallucinations. Fischman (1983) elaborated on this process and summarized the work of others who described this regressive transformation as the "concrete attitude." This attitude was defined as one in which the subject resorts to concrete sensory perceptions to comprehend and express certain situations, because of the impairment in conceptual thinking and abstraction.

As indicated earlier, hallucinations often accompany delusions during psychotic states, and may represent the concrete symbolic expression of delusional ideas that are seeking other routes of expression. The degree of the regressive transformation and the predominance of primary process seem to influence the choice of the symptom during psychosis. The emergence of hallucinations versus delusions may also be related to the degree of the cognitive limitations of the patient.

Modern psychodynamic views, such as the concepts presented by object relations theories, offer a different understanding of hallucinatory phenomena. Bion (1967) formulated the concept that early sensory impressions and perceptions constitute the early primitive elements of thoughts which he called "beta elements." He theorized that those elements predate the capacity for thinking itself, or what he called "an apparatus for thinking thoughts." He felt that beta elements represent early primitive elements of internalized bad objects which he also called "bizarre objects." He concluded that hallucinations occur as a result of projective identification, with the violent expulsion and projection of bizarre objects. When those elements are projected, they are experienced by the individual as existing in the external world and this forms the basis of a hallucination. Bion elaborated that beta elements occur when a baby is seriously frustrated and when wishful hallucination breaks down in the face of continued frustration. Thus, in an attempt to get rid of the unpleasant emotional state, these bad objects are evacuated in the form of primitive types of projections leading to hallucinatory experiences.

The psychodynamic theories outlined above offer some understanding of the underlying psychological factors involved in hallucinatory experiences, but they do not provide adequate explanation of the mechanism and etiology of these complicated phenomena.

PSYCHO-PHYSIOLOGICAL THEORIES

Ancient philosophers studied the hallucinatory phenomena and attempted to explain the mechanism of their occurrence. Although most of the thinking at those times focused on spiritual and philosophical explanations, some philosophers attempted to relate such experiences to physiologic mechanisms and anatomic loci. Plato (428–348 B.C.) believed that hallucinations arose in the liver, whereas rational thoughts and perceptions originated in the head. Aristotle (384–322 B.C.) believed that the heart was the major organ of mind where hallucinations occurred.

During the Middle Ages, some attention was given to notions of localized functions of the brain. This trend continued during the 17th and 18th centuries.

In the 19th century several physicians focused on the brain as the organ responsible for the occurrence of hallucinations and attempted to explain the phenomena utilizing physiological and anatomical concepts, more in line with our current knowledge of the structure and functions of the Central Nervous System. Before the turn of the century, Jackson (1932) proposed a major theory in an attempt to explain the hallucinatory phenomena. He formulated that the Central Nervous System is seen as having three evolutionary levels: the higher cortical level, the middle structures, which includes the basal ganglia; and the lower level, which includes the spinal cord. Jackson believed that hallucinations occur when the usual inhibitory influences of the uppermost level, i.e., the cerebral cortex, are impeded, leading to the release of middle-level activity, which takes the form of hallucinations. Thus, Jackson's model is one of dissociation leading to disinhibition and, consequently, the emergence of hallucinations.

Modern researchers have proposed further modifications of the dissociation and disinhibition theories of hallucinations. Marrazzi (1970) suggested that hallucination is an aberrant perception that can come about because of a dissociation of the new information arriving at the primary receiving cortical area from the past information stored in an association cortical area. He concluded that such dissociation is indicative of functional disintegration or failure of cerebral homeostasis. Marrazzi argued that such dissociative states occur not only in "functional" psychotic states, such as schizophrenia, but also in many organic states that may interfere with normal functioning of the brain, such as expanding brain tumors, as well as the ingestion of hallucinogenic drugs.

Fischer (1970) proposed a "sensory–motor ratio" theory focusing on a disequilibrium between the internal and the external sensory inputs to the Central Nervous System, leading to increased sensory awareness and decreased motor responsiveness. Consequently, he defined hallucinations as "intense sensory experiences with simultaneously inhibited or blocked intention and ability to verify those sensations through voluntary motor activity."

Slade (1976) hypothesized a four-factor theory of auditory hallucinations. The first factor involves the occurrence of internal emotional arousal in response to psychological stress. Such arousal interacts with the second factor which involves the hallucinatory predisposition threshold. This may raise the hallucinatory tendency above a certain level. If the degree of external stimulation (third factor) is not high enough to compete with the internal stimulation, the patient may consciously experience hallucinations. The fourth factor refers to the improvement of mood states as a consequence of the hallucination.

The role of internal arousal in relation to the mechanism of hallucinations was studied by other researchers. Cooklin et al. (1983) traced skin conductance in schizophrenic patients during periods of auditory hallucinations. They concluded that the onset of a hallucinatory period was associated with a substantial rise in the spontaneous fluctuation rate of skin conductance, an index of autonomic arousal. They were uncertain about whether arousal predisposes one to hallucinations or the onset of hallucinatory experience increases arousal level. Nevertheless, they concluded that internal arousal played some role in predisposing the person to hallucinatory activity.

A more comprehensive concept was presented by West (1962, 1975) who proposed the "perceptual release" theory. He suggested that the human brain is bombarded constantly by sensory stimuli of various kinds from the surrounding environment, as well as from within the brain itself. The brain selectively excludes from consciousness the majority of impulses that are irrelevant to attentiveness or otherwise not needed for environmental adaptation. According to the theory, the censorship mechanism in a normal subject can operate properly only if there is a constant flow of sensory impulses from the surrounding environment. Such a flow serves to inhibit earlier perceptions that are stored within the brain from emerging into consciousness. If the flow of sensory impulses is disturbed or absent, as in the case of prolonged periods of sensory deprivation, faulty synaptic transmission during toxic states, or excessive affect during "functional" psychosis, then the censorship mechanism is impaired. This impairment will allow the emergence of earlier perceptions or "traces" into consciousness, which will be reexperienced by the individual as hallucinations. West added that increased cortical arousal, which is usually induced by the diminution of sensory input, is an essential factor for this process to take place.

Other neurophysiological investigators have indicated that abnormal excitation of brain tissue may contribute to hallucinations. Penfield and Rasmussen (1950) reported the results of the experimental work that consisted of stimulating the exposed cerebral cortex of patients who had had neurologically uncontrolled epileptic seizures. Auditory and visual hallucinations of meaningful quality occurred only on stimulations of areas in or near the temporal lobe cortex. Penfield and his associates concluded that electrical stimulation of the temporal lobe cortex could, at times, activate records of previous experiences. Advances in neurosurgical techniques permitted stimulation of deeper structures of the brain. Jasper and Rasmussen (1958) inserted electrodes into deep structures of the temporal lobe and reported the occurrence of hallucinations or illusions in some patients. Winters (1975) concluded on the basis of several neuropharmacological studies in animals that the disorganization of sensory systems and perceptual abnormalities in hallucinations may result from states of hyperexcitation of the Central Nervous System.

Siegel and Jarvik (1975) proposed that the human mind can be viewed as an "information processing system" with sensory input and output. The system is responsible for scanning and screening information relating sensory input to mentation, and then integrating perception and mentation into action. They suggested that hallucinations occur when the integrative function of the system is compromised. In such instances, imagery is projected outside the subject and viewed as separate from the projector. Horowitz (1975) also proposed an information processing model. He argued that hallucinations are the final common pathway of various determinants in the information processing system that cause a subject erroneously to regard an image of internal origin as an external perception.

Other theories have proposed some involvement of the memory retrieval system in the mechanism of hallucinatory phenomena. The argument is based on similarities between dreams and hallucinations, and on the fact that memory traces may constitute building blocks of dreams. There has not been any clinical research to support such theories. However, it is clear that memory traces and unconscious material are closely linked to hallucinations.

Some researchers (Mintz & Alpert, 1972) have suggested that hallucinations occur in certain people because of enhanced vividness capacity. However, Starker and Jolin (1982) challenged that theory and found clinical evidence to support an imagery deficit model in hallucinating schizophrenic patients. Richardson and Divyo (1980) compared a group of alcoholic hallucinators with a group of alcoholic non-hallucinators and found that the former group showed an impaired ability to make clear perceptual-conceptual distinction (i.e., boundary confusion).

Green (1987) proposed that hallucinations represent verbal activity that occurs in the non-dominant hemisphere. He added that schizophrenic patients may suffer from defective information transfer between the two cerebral hemispheres. Bentall and Slade (1985) compared a group of schizophrenic hallucinators to another group of schizophrenic non-hallucinators and found that hallucinators have a greater tendency to believe under some conditions that stimuli are real even when they are not. They indicated that cognitive ability to assess reality is involved in the mechanism of hallucinatory experience. Zigler and Levine (1983) have reported that hallucinating patients were at a lower developmental level than delusional patients, emphasizing the role of cognitive limitation of patients who are predisposed to hallucinations.

The similarities between hallucinations and dreams have been known for a long time. Hartmann (1975) formulated a neurophysiological mechanism to explain both phenomena which, he felt, lie on a continuum. He suggested that an inhibitory factor, psychologically related to the function of "reality testing" and physiologically mediated by ascending cortical noradrenergic systems, prevents the emergence of both hallucinations and dreams into the waking state. When this inhibitory mechanism is disrupted by physiological or biochemical factors, hallucinations and dreams are experienced.

The correlation between hallucination and REM sleep was investigated by Dement et al. (1969), who proposed that a defective serotonin gating mechanism allowed some phasic events of REM sleep to intrude into the waking state. They noticed that Pontine-geniculate-occipital (PGO) waves, which are normally confined to electroencephalographic tracings during REM sleep, emerged into the non-REM waking states and seemed to coincide with hallucinatory-like behavior in animals. Although these findings were inconclu-

sive, the correlation between hallucinations and REM sleep remains significant. Further evidence to support such correlation is derived from the observations that transcontinental air travel may induce hallucinations. Snyder (1983)
hypothesized that altered sleep-stage architecture with shifts in REM onset
and periodicity may be etiologically related to hallucinations.

More recent research studies have investigated regional cerebral blood
flow during hallucinations. Mathew et al. (1982) reported that in some cases
of hallucinating patients there is reduced blood flow to several postcentral
cerebral regions during hallucinations, whereas in others there is increased
temporoparietal blood flow. A recent report by Hemmingsen et al. (1988)
indicated that greater cerebral blood flow was significantly correlated with
visual hallucinations and agitation during the acute withdrawal reaction in
patients with delirium tremens.

Cerebral glucography utilizing Positron Emission Tomography (PET) has
been employed in investigating hallucinatory phenomena. Buchsbaum et al.
(1982) suggested that schizophrenic patients have a greater glucose uptake
by the auditory areas and the temporal lobe during auditory hallucinations.

Green and Preston (1981) reported that auditory hallucinations in schizophrenic patients may be accompanied by vocalizations that are observed to
occur concurrently with hallucinations. The content of such vocalizations
corresponds to what the voices are reported to have said. They noticed that
such vocalizations could be increased to an intelligible level by the use of
auditory feedback. More recently, Bick and Kinsbourne (1987) reported that
in some hallucinating schizophrenic patients, the voices they heard went
away when they undertook a maneuver that precluded subvocalizations,
such as opening the mouth. They suggested that "auditory hallucinations
may be projections of schizophrenic patients' verbal thoughts, subvocalized
due to deficient cerebral cortical inhibition."

Several reports have noted functional and anatomical cerebral asymmetry
associated with hallucinations in schizophrenic patients. The significance of
these findings remains unclear.

Here too, we find that the psychophysiological theories may provide
partial explanation for the hallucinatory phenomena from various aspects
and viewpoints, but none has yet been integrated into a comprehensive
pathophysiological concept that can adequately explain the mechanism of
hallucinations.

NEUROCHEMICAL THEORIES

It is widely known that brain functions are mediated via neurotransmitters
and through biochemical processes affecting various receptors and synapses.
Research in the field of psychopharmacology and molecular neurobiology has
accelerated in the past decade and has shed some light on the mechanisms of
brain functions, as well as pathological phenomena affecting the brain, includ-

ing hallucinations. Furthermore, the regular occurrence of hallucinations as symptoms of nonpsychiatric medical conditions and as side effects of many medications has stimulated researchers to investigate the biochemical aspects of hallucinatory phenomena.

Kraepelin was the first to attempt a systematic study of the phenomenology of mental illness by utilizing chemically induced psychoses as a model for "endogenous psychosis." Several other researchers employed various hallucinogenic agents, such as mescaline, for the same purpose. Later LSD was used as an experimental tool for inducing psychosis in attempts to uncover the biochemical mechanisms leading to psychosis (Fischman, 1983). It was subsequently concluded by Hollister (1968) and others that the drug-induced and schizophrenic states were markedly different. The predominant type of hallucinations induced by drugs was visual, whereas hallucinations in schizophrenic states were mainly auditory. Furthermore, delusions were rare in drug-induced psychotic states, and there was no thought disorder or speech disorder. However, many writers found several similarities between schizophrenic states and drug-induced psychotic states, including the hallucinatory experiences. In this regard, some studies have shown consistently that visual hallucinations are more common than auditory hallucinations among schizophrenics in the Near East and Africa (Fischman, 1983). After a lengthy review by Fischman (1983), it was concluded that the two states, though they may be different, still share certain fundamental properties. In any event, this type of work set the stage for further biological research in which several neurotransmitters were identified to be involved in the mechanism of hallucinatory phenomena.

Among the neurotransmitters that are believed to be responsible for producing hallucinatory symptoms, dopamine seems to play a major role. The dopamine hypothesis (Fischman, 1983) was based upon two major findings: (1) Pharmacological agents that decrease dopaminergic activity have antipsychotic properties, and (2) Drugs that increase dopaminergic activity produce psychotic states that are virtually indistinguishable from schizophrenia. It is well known that treatment of Parkinson's disease with L-DOPA preparations may induce psychosis, mainly a hallucinatory syndrome. It is believed that such an action is a result of the drug's direct dopaminergic effect. Nausieda et al. (1983) suggested that L-DOPA produced hallucinations either because of the progressive dementia that occurs in the course of Parkinson's disease, which tends to predispose the patient to this side effect, or because of the direct effect of the drug. It is also well known that antipsychotic medications that block central dopamine activity alleviate the hallucinatory symptoms, a connection that points toward the involvement of dopamine in the mechanism of hallucinations. Further evidence in support of such involvement is derived from the observation that d-amphetamine, an indirect dopamine agonist, induces psychosis and hallucinations in some people.

Although the exact mechanism by which dopamine contributes to the production of hallucinations is still unclear, the role of this major neurotransmitter in mediating psychotic processes and hallucinatory symptoms is indisputable.

The involvement of serotonin has also been considered in the biochemistry of hallucinations. It is believed that low central levels of serotonin might be an important factor. In fact, a number of hallucinogenic drugs, such as Lysergide (LSD), Mescaline, Psilocin, Dimethyltryptamine (DMT) and other related preparations appear to act, at least in part, by blocking central serotonergic receptors (Nauseida et al., 1983). Furthermore, it is known that certain hallucinogenic drugs such as LSD, DMT, Psilocin share the indole nucleus, which is also found in the neurotransmitter serotonin. This shared nucleus may be the basis for the mechanism by which hallucinogens exert their serotonergic inhibitory effect. Amphetamines, which have been known to act via the dopaminergic system, seem to affect the serotoneregic system as well. It has been suggested that chronic administration of amphetamine leads to decrease in both serotonin and 5-HIAA levels which leads to hallucinatory experience (Fischman, 1983).

Despite the clear evidence of the serotonin involvement in the hallucinatory phenomena, some studies have failed to find a consistent relationship between depression of serotonergic neurons and behavior (Trulson & Jacobs, 1979a). However, it remains clear that serotonin plays a significant role in the biochemical mechanism of hallucinations.

Some reports have suggested that cholinergic transmission may also be involved in the hallucinatory process. Goetz et al. (1982) reported that manipulation of either dopaminergic drugs or anticholinergic drugs in the course of treating patients with Parkinson's disease could precipitate or relieve hallucinations. They concluded that dopaminergic/cholinergic systems are reciprocally active in the pathophysiology of long-term, drug-induced hallucinatory states in certain patients.

Several other biochemical mechanisms have been suggested to be involved in the hallucinatory phenomena. Domino and Ruffing (1982) suggested a role for the opioid receptors in the behavioral response to hallucinogens. They observed that opioid antagonists can potentiate the behavioral effects of both DMT and LSD in rats. Gunne et al. (1977) had concluded earlier that changes in endorphins levels were in part responsible for symptoms in schizophrenia, including hallucinations.

Another area of neurochemical interest has been the role of monoamine oxidase (MAO) in hallucinatory experiences. Some studies have noted an association between low platelets MAO activity and hallucinations in schizophrenics (Meltzer et al., 1980). Brandys and Yehuda (1983) argued that hallucinogens have an inhibitory effect on the MAOs.

Again, in the biochemical arena, we find a number of theories and research findings that may shed light on some aspects of the mechanisms involved in causing the hallucinatory symptoms, but none of these theories seems to offer an adequate explanation.

SUMMARY

The psychodynamic, psychophysiological, and neurochemical aspects discussed above seem to provide very interesting and convincing data in support of various theories and hypotheses. However, they do not offer an integrated comprehensive mechanism to account for the etiology and pathogenesis of hallucinations. Such an integrated approach will be discussed later in this book and will consider several relevant factors including biological vulnerability and psychological influences.

6 ═

Hallucinations in Psychiatric Disorders

Hallucinations occur in a wide variety of psychiatric disorders, ranging from schizophrenia to certain personality disorders. The clinical presentation of the hallucinatory experiences with regard to their type, complexity, and content may vary from one condition to another, though they still cannot be considered pathognomonic of any given disorder. Furthermore, it should be emphasized that the long-standing notion that hallucinations are to be equated with schizophrenia is clearly unfounded. In the following few pages, the attempt is made to review hallucinatory symptoms as they present in various psychiatric disorders.

SCHIZOPHRENIA

Hallucinations represent one of the major psychotic symptoms of schizophrenic disorders. The most common type of hallucination in schizophrenia is auditory. Such hallucinations are usually formed and complex. Most characteristically, two voices talk about and discuss the patient in the third person. They may debate in an approving or antagonistic manner, or they may command the patient to act in a certain way. Command hallucinations represent unconscious wishes of behaving in a certain way that may not be acceptable to the ego on a conscious level. These hallucinations have generally been considered to be serious because, in some instances, the patient may act in response to them and proceed with bizarre, destructive, or suicidal behavior. Such patients may require some form of observation or close psychiatric attention to ameliorate the symptoms as quickly as possible. However, a recent study reported by Hellerstein et al. (1987) indicated that patients with command hallucinations were not significantly different from patients without command hallucinations on demographic and behavioral variables, such as suicidal ideation, suicidal behavior, or assaultiveness. They concluded that command hallucinations alone may not imply greater risk for acute, life-threatening behavior. Despite this conclusion, it is advisable that clinicians continue to regard such patients as at higher risk for destructive behavior and to provide special precautions and a more aggressive treatment approach to prevent the emergence of such behavior.

It is important to mention here that auditory hallucinations in the condition known as alcoholic hallucinosis may resemble to a large extent, the auditory hallucinations of schizophrenia, and may even have a commanding nature. Hallucinations associated with alcoholism will be discussed in Chapter 7.

Schizophrenic patients often report hearing the voices of God and the devil. They sometimes hear the voices of relatives or neighbors. Frequently, patients can neither recognize nor understand the voices. The voices may be heard as coming from inside the head or from outside. Such distinction does not seem to reflect significant clinical difference among schizophrenic patients. However, it is felt that patients who acknowledge that the voices are coming from within their head, or that they are hearing their own thoughts, may have less disrupted ego functions, and more insight into the unreality of their experiences (Koehler, 1979). In addition, schizophrenic patients of both sexes can hear both male and female voices. Gruber et al. (1984) investigated the laterality of hallucinations in a mixed group of patients. They reported that some patients were able to describe the voices they hear as coming from the left side of the head or from the right side. Still, in the majority of patients, no such localization was possible. They concluded that subjects who heard voices on the right side were found to be significantly more depressed than others. It should be noted here that in clinical practice, no attention is usually paid to the laterality of auditory hallucinations, and the significance of such an observation remains to be seen.

The content of auditory hallucinations provides an important tool for understanding the psychodynamic issues that are involved in the illness. The voices may be friendly and benign. They may comment on what the patient is doing and what is going on around him or her. However, the voices may be very hostile or threatening. A patient who feels inadequate and wishes to be accepted and approved of by others may hear voices telling him that he is "the greatest," or that he has been chosen to save the world. A similar patient with feelings of inferiority may hear voices making condescending remarks about her. In the first example, the commending hallucinatory experience serves to fulfill the patient's unconscious wishes to be superior and to be accepted by others; whereas in the second example, the critical voices represent the concrete symbolic projection of her feelings of her negative self image. Usually the content of the hallucinatory experience is of the same nature as the content of the delusions and thinking in general, or they are, at least, psychodynamically related.

As indicated earlier, auditory hallucinations may be difficult to recognize or understand. In fact, less complex, unformed auditory hallucinations are reported frequently by schizophrenic patients. Some patients may simply hear their names being called, or they may hear simple words such as "no" or "stop." At times, the words may be mumbled or incomplete. Some patients report hearing music or whistling. Occasionally schizophrenic patients report hearing laughter, whispers, footsteps, humming, knocking on the door, bells, and other sounds. It is important to mention that such unformed, simple auditory hallucinations are more characteristic of organic psychotic states than schizophrenia. However, they are definitely present in some schizophrenic patients.

Visual hallucinations occur less frequently than do auditory hallucinations in schizophrenic patients, but they are not uncommon. Visual hallucinations within the course of schizophrenic disorder occur at all times, day or night. They are usually formed and complex. Patients report seeing people, pictures, animals, and other objects. Objects are seen nearby, clearly defined, usually in colors and life size, and sometimes moving. Some patients describe seeing events taking place in front of them.

Occasionally, visual hallucinations in schizophrenia are less formed. In such instances, patients may report seeing fuzzy images, circles, lines, or flashes of light. Such experiences are more characteristic of organic mental disorders or drug-induced psychosis. However, in cases of organic etiology, visual hallucinations are more intense at nighttime, in darkened surroundings, or when the eyes are closed, in contrast to the visual hallucinations of schizophrenia which do not change by environmental manipulation. In addition, visual hallucinations of schizophrenia, and other "functional" psychotic states, appear suddenly and without prodromata in a psychological setting of intense affective need or delusional preoccupation.

Visual hallucinations are usually experienced in addition to auditory hallucinations in schizophrenic patients. However, some studies have suggested that visual hallucinations may represent the main modality of hallucinations in schizophrenia. Fischman (1983) reported the results of several international studies of schizophrenic populations. He indicated that such studies have shown consistently that visual hallucinations are more common than auditory hallucinations among schizophrenics in the Near East and in Africa. Furthermore, he indicated that close temporal studies of hallucinations in Western patients suggest that only recently has the frequency of auditory hallucinations exceeded that of visual hallucinations. Other writers have reported similar findings. Small et al. (1966) found that visual and other nonauditory hallucinations were fairly common among schizophrenic patients. The authors reported that visual hallucinations occurred in 30 percent of the 50 schizophrenic patients who participated in their study. Jansson (1969) also reported similar findings indicating that visual hallucinations occurred in almost half of the 83 suspected schizophrenics who had been investigated in his study.

The content of visual hallucinations reflects the underlying psychodynamic issues. The visual hallucinations are usually consistent with the auditory hallucinations and with the delusional thinking. A schizophrenic patient who is religiously preoccupied and hears the voice of God talking to her, may see the image of Christ outside the window, or may simply see crosses on the walls. Another patient who believes that aliens have landed may report hearing a strange language spoken by little hairless people who are walking around. Some schizophrenic patients are observed carrying out conversations with hallucinated people as if they were with them in the same room. In the examples described above, we see that the visual hallucinations, like auditory hallucinations, serve to further express and symbolize delusional beliefs.

Tactile hallucinations, also known as "haptic hallucinations," are reported less frequently in schizophrenia. Here, too, the hallucinatory experience provides a further concrete channel to express the underlying psychodynamic situation or need. A schizophrenic patient may report a feeling of electricity passing through his body. Another patient may feel an external power is holding her and controlling her movements. Occasionally, tactile hallucinations may accompany bizarre sexual delusions in schizophrenic patients. For example, one patient felt that he had a continuous erection that was forced on him by a condom manufacturer in order to use him in its advertising campaign (Walker & Cavenar, 1983). However, the occurrence of tactile hallucinations should alert the clinician to look for organic causes such as delirium tremens, or cocaine and amphetamine intoxication states. Tactile hallucinations are rarely reported independent of other forms of hallucinations in schizophrenic patients. Typically, tactile hallucinations accompany auditory or visual hallucinations.

Olfactory hallucinations and gustatory hallucinations also occur in schizophrenia. They may be experienced independently or in conjunction with other types of hallucinations. Most often, they come as part of a delusional system. The odors are usually unpleasant. A patient with somatic delusions may hallucinate offensive odors emanating from her own body. Sometimes, patients may report smelling smoke or perfumes. A patient hallucinated a female figure and smelled her perfume. A delusional patient who believed that someone was trying to poison him, hallucinated the taste of arsenic in his food.

As olfactory hallucinations and gustatory hallucinations are particularly present in organic conditions such as temporal lobe lesions and uncinate fits, all patients with such symptoms, including schizophrenics, should be evaluated appropriately to rule out these conditions.

In addition to the different types of hallucinations described above, schizophrenic patients may report more complex hallucinatory experiences. Cenesthetic hallucinations refer to deep visceral sensations that cannot be perceived by normal individuals, yet are felt by some schizophrenic patients (Solomon & Patch, 1974). For example, a patient might report feeling a burning sensation inside her brain, or feeling the blood flowing into her heart. These hallucinations are relatively rare.

BIPOLAR DISORDERS

In manic depressive disorders accompanied by psychotic features, hallucinatory experiences may resemble to a great extent the hallucinations of schizophrenia. In fact, in some instances, the differential diagnosis between bipolar disorder with psychotic features and other psychotic disorders may be extremely difficult. This is particularly true when the clinical presentation is evaluated on a cross-sectional basis (Asaad, 1988). The most frequent type of hallucinations in affective disorders is auditory, followed by the visual type, as is the case with schizophrenia (Goodwin et al., 1971). Unlike auditory hallucinations of schizophrenia, the auditory hallucinations of mania are transient, are of shorter duration, and usually are confined to the acute state of the manic syndrome. The hallucinations are usually clear voices of people talking to the patient or about him or her. Sometimes the hallucinations are less formed, and may be limited to simple sounds or music. Here, too, the content of the hallucinations reflects the underlying psychodynamic situations and needs. Most often, the hallucinations in affective disorders are mood-congruent, and are closely related to the delusional beliefs held by the patient. A manic patient with elated mood and inflated self-esteem heard the voice of God telling him that he was the greatest man on earth and that he was chosen by God to save the world. Another manic female patient who was sexually preoccupied reported receiving phone calls from men propositioning her and inviting her to have sex with them. Less commonly, the content of the hallucinations has no apparent relationship to the predominant mood (mood-incongruent) (DSM-III-R, 1987).

Visual hallucinations also are found in manic states with psychotic features. They usually occur with auditory hallucinations, but they may occur alone. The are usually formed, mood-congruent, and express the psychodynamic conflict of the patient. A sexually preoccupied, manic male patient had hallucinations of naked women during which he masturbated repeatedly.

Other types of hallucinations do occur in manic syndromes as well. Tactile hallucinations involving sexual stimulation of external genitalia have been reported by some patients. Olfactory and gustatory hallucinations are less frequent in manic states, but they can occur in some patients. A patient with a history of bipolar disorder reported smelling fumes in her car and at home during every manic episode she experienced.

MAJOR DEPRESSION

When major depression is complicated by psychotic features, hallucinations may be present as part of the clinical picture. However, they are usually transient and not elaborate. Typically, the hallucinations are clearly consistent with the predominant mood (mood-congruent). Less frequently, they are mood-incongruent (DSM-III-R, 1987). Auditory hallucinations are more common than other modalities. Usually, patients hear voices accusing them of sins never committed in reality. Occasionally, the voices may command patients to kill themselves. Patients are usually delusional and firmly believe that they have committed unforgivable sins and that they do not deserve to live. Visual and other types of hallucinations are also reported in psychotic depression.

SCHIZOAFFECTIVE DISORDERS

Hallucinatory experience in the course of schizoaffective disorders is quite similar to that of schizophrenia and affective disorders discussed above. Hallucinations are usually chronic, elaborate, and of the auditory type. They are frequently consistent with predominant mood, but mood-incongruent hallucinations are not uncommon. In addition, visual, tactile, olfactory, and gustatory hallucinations are reported.

SCHIZOPHRENIFORM DISORDERS

Hallucinations in schizophreniform disorders are usually similar to those of schizophrenia, and all material presented under schizophrenic hallucinations may be applied to the syndrome with the exception of duration. By definition, the duration of the symptoms in schizophreniform disorder is from one month to six months (DSM-III-R, 1987).

BRIEF REACTIVE PSYCHOSIS

Hallucinations in the course of brief reactive psychosis occur in response to an identifiable stressor usually in patients with a histrionic personality. Other symptoms, such as delusions, derealizations and bizarre behavior often occur. Hallucinations tend to be more visual and dreamlike, and the patient usually demonstrates an expansive and effervescent affect (Walker & Cavenar, 1983). The duration of symptoms is generally less than one month.

DELUSIONAL DISORDERS

It is unusual to encounter hallucinatory experiences in the course of delusional disorders, formerly known as paranoid disorders. However, in rare cases, transient nonprominent auditory or visual hallucinations may be experienced by some patients (DSM-III-R, 1987). The content of the hallucinations is usually consistent with the nature of the delusional material. In addition, the patient generally exhibits a full range of appropriate affect. The degree of the insight toward the unreality of the hallucinatory experience is variable. A patient who believed that a famous singer was in love with her began to experience hearing his songs. She was convinced that only she could hear the songs because he was singing them just for her.

PERSONALITY DISORDERS

Patients with borderline personality disorder are known to undergo transient "micropsychotic" episodes during which they may experience hallucinations of various modalities. The experience is very brief and the patient is usually able to appreciate the unreality of the perceptions.

Patients with schizotypal personality disorder rarely present with true hallucinations. Rather, they report unusual perceptual experiences such as sensing the presence of a special force or person not actually present. Illusions are reported as well (DSM-III-R, 1987). Some patients with schizoid personality disorder may report hallucinatory experiences on rare occasions.

POST-TRAUMATIC STRESS DISORDER

The most prominent clinical features of post-traumatic stress disorder include: reexperiencing the trauma; numbed responsiveness, or reduced involvement with the external world; and a variety of other depressive, autonomic, and cognitive symptoms.

A definite group of patients with PTSD report pseudo or real auditory and visual hallucinations. Mueser and Butler (1987) studied a group of veterans with post-traumatic stress disorder and found that those veterans who had higher combat exposure and sustained more intense post-traumatic stress disorder symptoms experienced auditory hallucinations in addition to other symptoms. In such instances, patients report hearing voices related to their traumatic experiences. Sometimes the voices tell patients to kill themselves. Waldfogel and Mueser (1988) reported the case of a veteran who suffered from PTSD that developed following a sexual assault, and who experienced auditory hallucinations and paranoid delusions. Although the patient met the DSM-III-R diagnostic criteria for schizophrenia, the authors concluded that the hallucinations and the delusions had been induced by PTSD, especially as the symptoms did not respond to antipsychotic medications. They added that the patient responded very well to imaginal flooding therapy, with sustained improvement.

Siegel (1984) reported that visual hallucinations occurred in people subjected to life threatening stress, such as hostage situations or rape. Victims frequently experienced auditory, visual, or tactile hallucinations as recurrent flashbacks in the course of their post-traumatic stress disorder.

Severe states of anxiety may be associated with hallucinations. Lukianowicz (1969) discussed the case of a child who was subjected to a series of life stresses and frightening events. The child started experiencing auditory hallucinations consisting of voices telling her that her mother would leave. In the dark, she also experienced visual hallucinations of dead people and crashed cars.

DISSOCIATIVE DISORDERS

Dissociative disorders involve sudden, temporary alterations in consciousness, identity, or motor behavior. Symptoms of amnesia, fugue states, and depersonalization experiences are common. Dissociative states serve as a defense against unconscious conflicts that may be on the verge of emerging into consciousness with resultant anxiety. It is widely held that dissociative phenomena are more common in persons with histrionic personality organization.

Hallucinations have been reported to occur during dissociative states in certain people. The most common type of hallucinations in such instances is visual. However, other types of hallucinations may occur as well. Kessler (1972) discussed dissociative hallucinations in children. He suggested that such hallucinations involve several different mechanisms, such as repression, displacement, and projection. He added that these hallucinations serve the purpose of creating a distance between the self and the source of the conflict. A patient with a history of conflicts concerning her sexuality reported experiencing dissociative states during which her deceased father would appear in front of her and tell her that she was a "bad girl." Dissociative experiences in this context are closely related to trance states and hypnosis in the sense that they represent states of altered level of consciousness that allow unconscious material to become readily available to conscious awareness. Depersonalization and derealization occur frequently in dissociative states as well.

Goodwin et al. (1971) investigated eight patients with the diagnosis of "hysteria." Their sample included women with histories of chronic polysymptomatic illness in the absence of a known medical disease. They found that seven patients reported hallucinatory experience of some kind. Four of them experienced hallucinations in more than three modalities. Five patients were aware of the unreality of the experience. In fact, it is appropriate to raise the question here whether the hallucinatory phenomena experienced by patients during dissociative states or in the "hysterical" syndrome are in fact true hallucinations. It is probably more accurate to refer to these experiences as pseudohallucinations (Asaad & Shapiro, 1986).

McKegney (1967, 1987) viewed some hallucinations as conversion symptoms representing a revival of experiences that occurred in the past at the time of satisfying relationships. Such patients appeared to hallucinate under psychological stress.

Related to the disorders mentioned above, is the condition known as "hysterical psychosis," also referred to as "pseudopsychosis." In this condition, the patient appears to suddenly lapse into a psychotic state characterized by hallucinations and delusions without the thought disorder or mood disorder. These psychotic symptoms have close association with underlying psychological factors, and, in many ways, are considered analogous to the physical symptoms in the course of conversion disorders (Bishop & Holt, 1980).

Multiple personality disorder is an entity related to the dissociative phenomena. Various types of hallucinations have been reported in the course of multiple personality syndrome.

SUMMARY

Hallucinations can occur in almost any psychiatric condition, including psychotic disorders, mood disorders, anxiety disorders, and personality disorders. Hallucinations of schizophrenia and other "functional" psychotic states tend to be auditory and of a complex nature. However, other types of hallucinations, as well as simple forms of hallucinations are not uncommon. When they occur in the course of anxiety disorders, dissociative states, or personality disorders, hallucinations are usually brief and are recognized by the individual as being unreal. Differential diagnosis is discussed in Chapter 16.

7

Hallucinations Associated with Alcoholism

Various types of hallucinations are described in association with certain clinical conditions related to alcoholism. Such hallucinatory symptoms may be experienced independently or in addition to other psychiatric and physical symptoms that occur in the course of organic mental disorders precipitated by alcohol withdrawal or long-term abuse.

BIOLOGICAL CONSIDERATIONS

Alcohol is known to have a depressant effect on the central nervous system similar to that of anesthetic agents. It is believed that alcohol acts initially on the reticular formation, leading to increased excitability and mild euphoria. Later it exerts its toxic effects directly on the cortical neurons. Withdrawal from alcohol can lead to series of episodes that include seizures, hallucinations, and delirium tremens. Wernicke's encephalopathy and Korsakoff's psychosis are believed to develop as a result of nutritional deficiencies that may be associated with alcohol consumption (Lishman, 1987).

The exact mechanism leading to hallucinatory phenomena occurring in the course of various syndromes associated with alcoholism is unknown. However, it is clear that hallucinations in these conditions are organic in nature and probably result from underlying physiological and neurochemical changes. Psychological and cultural factors are likely to influence the hallucinatory experiences as well.

Contrary to previously held beliefs, there is no evidence that schizophrenia predisposes to the development of alcohol hallucinosis (DSM-III-R, 1987).

Saravay and Pardes (1970) postulated that certain sounds and noises heard by patients with alcohol withdrawal psychosis are produced by muscular contractions of the middle ear and are not indicative of psychosis. They proposed that these sounds should not be considered true hallucinations. Such views are not supported by adequate research or clinical evidence.

Fasullo and Lupo (1973) studied the psychopathological aspects of delirium tremens. They suggested that an increase in REM sleep may influence the production of visual hallucinations in delirium tremens. The increased REM sleep during delirium tremens is believed to represent a rebound reaction due to withdrawal from alcohol which normally suppresses REM sleep.

Ballenger and Post (1978) proposed that repeated heavy administration of alcohol over prolonged periods of time may have "kindling" effects on the brain. They hypothesized that intoxication and withdrawal are accompanied by minor dysrhythmia in the brain. Limbic system hyperirritability accompanying each episode of withdrawal is likely to increase over time through the kindling process and to spread widely in subcortical structures. They concluded that long-term changes in neuronal excitability may, accordingly, underlie the progressive escalation of withdrawal symptoms starting with tremors, then seizures, and ultimately leading into delirium tremens.

Shen (1985) reviewed the records of 1,911 alcoholic patients and found significant correlation between the onset of hallucinations and the presence of nausea and vomiting in these patients. He suggested that there may be a potential link between the occurrence of nausea and vomiting and the onset of hallucinations in alcohol intoxication/withdrawal states.

Branchey et al. (1985) studied plasma amino acids of alcoholics. They found that patients with a history of hallucinations had significantly lower plasma tryptophan ratios in comparison to those patients without such a history. In addition, alcoholics with hallucinations had significantly high plasma tyrosine plus phenylalanine ratios as compared to alcoholics without hallucinations. They concluded that amino acid abnormalities believed to result in decreased brain serotonin and increased brain dopamine may render certain individuals more vulnerable to hallucinatory experiences. Their data suggest that amino acid abnormalities, which are common in alcoholics, may modify serotonin and dopamine pathways in such individuals, and eventually result in hallucinatory phenomena.

A recent report by Hemmingsen et al. (1988) indicated that regional cerebral blood flow was increased and seemed to significantly correlate with visual hallucinations and agitation observed in patients during alcohol withdrawal syndrome. They concluded that delirium tremens and related clinical states represent a type of acute brain syndrome, mainly characterized by central nervous system hyperexcitability.

CLINICAL SYNDROMES

Alcohol Withdrawal Delirium (Delirium Tremens)

This syndrome usually begins on the second or third day after the cessation or reduction of drinking, but may have its onset as early as one day or as late as one week after abstinence (Asaad & Shapiro, 1986). Symptoms include clouding of consciousness, disorientation, tremulousness, agitation, and autonomic hyperactivity. Vivid hallucinations that may be visual, auditory, or tactile are common. The first episode of this disorder usually occurs following five to 15 years of heavy drinking. The presence of a concomitant physical illness seems to predispose to this syndrome (DSM-III-R, 1987).

The onset is usually sudden, and often at night. The early signs of perceptual disturbances involve hyperexcitability, startling, and vivid nightmares. Transient illusions and hallucinations follow, accompanied by intense anxiety. As the physical condition deteriorates, psychotic symptoms intensify. Illusions become more pronounced. Spots on the wall may be mistaken for insects, and cracks in the ceiling may be seen as snakes. Visual hallucinations predominate the clinical presentation. They typically consist of fleeting, recurrent, and changeable images that compulsively hold the patient's attention. Rats, snakes, and other small animals are reported to be seen by patients, and can appear in colorful and vivid forms. Objects, animals, and persons are frequently seen reduced in size. Lishman (1987) described visual hallucinations experienced by patients during delirium tremens. He observed a patient "who followed intently, and with excited comments, a game of football performed for half an hour on end by two teams of normal-colored miniature elephants in a corner of his room." Other visual hallucinations may be in full size and involve seeing faces, or fantastic scenes. The psychological and cultural factors seem to influence the content of hallucinatory experiences. A patient who works as a station master reported seeing trains rapidly approaching him. A factory worker hallucinated his work bench in front of him and went through his work activities with excitement (Lishman, 1987). Visual hallucinations of delirium tremens may be very difficult to differentiate from visual hallucinations of any other acute organic brain condition.

Tactile hallucinations are fairly common in alcoholic withdrawal delirium. They are experienced typically as small animals crawling over the skin. This condition is also known as "formication." Tactile hallucinations of similar nature also occur during cocaine and amphetamine intoxication.

Auditory hallucinations are less frequent than are visual and tactile hallucinations in alcohol withdrawal delirium. When they occur, they are commonly of a threatening or persecutory nature. These hallucinations should be differentiated from auditory hallucinations of psychotic states, such as schizophrenia, and from those of alcoholic hallucinosis which occur in states of clear consciousness. Unlike schizophrenic auditory hallucinations and alcoholic hallucinosis, these hallucinations occur only during the delirious state that results from alcoholic withdrawal, and are accompanied by changes in the vital signs. This differentiation is important, since the management of each condition is different as outlined below.

Alcohol withdrawal delirium should be recognized and treated immediately as a medical emergency due to the serious complications that can follow, which include possible mortality. In the majority of cases, this disorder lasts less than three days. With proper management, recovery is usually complete and without complications. However, about 15 percent of all cases of delirium tremens go on to become Korsakoff's syndrome (chronic alcohol psychosis) characterized by memory impairment, disorientation, and particularly, confabulation (Linn, 1985). This may occur, especially, when Wernicke's encephalopathy had been present but went unnoticed during the acute stage of the delirium tremens. Treatment should be carried out in the hospital with prompt fluid replacement and adequate sedation. The patient should be kept in a well lit room with a staff member present in order to prevent accidental injuries that may result from agitation and confusion. Some patients have jumped out of the hospital windows during delirious states. Vital signs should be monitored frequently. Patients should be started on benzodiazepines immediately followed by a proper detoxification regimen. A small dose of a high potency antipsychotic medication is essential to control the hallucinatory symptom and to reduce the patient's agitation. The dosage can be titrated upwards or downwards according to the clinical response. Finally, vitamin supplementation is essential. Thiamine hydrochloride as well as multivitamins should be given. All medical complications need to be addressed and treated appropriately.

Alcohol Hallucinosis

Alcohol hallucinosis is different from delirium tremens and presents mainly with auditory hallucinations that persist after a person has recovered from symptoms of delirium tremens, and is no longer in the state of clouded consciousness. Usually the symptoms appear within the first 48 hours of cessation of alcohol intake, but may be delayed for as long as one or two weeks following abstinence (Asaad & Shapiro, 1986). In some cases, the hallucinations may begin when there is a drop in blood alcohol level toward the end of an extended period of drinking. Thus, they may appear first as part of an alcohol withdrawal delirium, and then persist after the delirious state is finished and the sensorium has completely cleared (Kaplan & Sadock, 1985).

The age of onset is around forty years old. However, episodes have been reported in people in their early to mid-twenties. The disorder is apparently four times more common in males than in females. Typically, its first appearance follows ten years or more of heavy drinking (DSM-III-R, 1987).

Hallucinations may begin as buzzing, mumbling, or crackling sounds and progress into vivid accusatory hallucinations posing threats to the patient or his or her family (Surawicz, 1980). The hallucinations are more prominent at night. When the voices are malicious and threatening, the patient may respond with fear and apprehension. Patients may need to be protected against injuring themselves or others in an effort to avoid the consequences of the threats made by the voices. Occasionally, the hallucinatory content may be benign and leave the person undisturbed. The voices may address the person directly, but more often they discuss him or her in the third person. Command hallucinations are also common. Visual hallucinations may occur as part of alcohol hallucinosis as well (DSM-III-R, 1987).

Most often hallucinations last for only a few hours or a few days, but in about 10 percent of patients hallucinations last weeks or months, becoming chronic in rare cases. With the evolution of the chronic form, which may be recognized as early as a week after onset, the patient may calm down, resigning him- or herself to the persisting hallucinations. Other psychotic symptoms such as ideas of reference and other poorly systematized persecutory delusions may become prominent. Occasionally, vague and illogical thinking, tangential association, and inappropriate affect develop, making the clinical presentation virtually indistinguishable from schizophrenia (DSM-III-R, 1987).

It is important to note here that the voices may command the patient to do things against his or her will, and their compelling quality may be such that the patient is driven to a suicidal attempt or to some episode of bizarre behavior (Lishman, 1987).

The course of this illness is still unclear, but it is generally believed that the chronic form is more likely to develop from repeated episodes of the disorder in persons with histories of heavy alcohol ingestion and who apparently have alcohol dependence.

Alcohol hallucinosis usually responds well to antipsychotic medications. Occasionally, ECT may be needed to terminate the attack abruptly in those cases which persist beyond a few weeks.

Wernicke's Encephalopathy

Wernicke's encephalopathy is believed to represent the acute neuropsychiatric reaction to severe thiamine deficiency. Alcoholism is an important, but not exclusive, cause of the disorder. Several other conditions are known to cause Wernicke's encephalopathy, including: carcinoma of the stomach, pregnancy, toxemia, pernicious anemia, vomiting, diarrhea, and dietary deficiency. The syndrome starts abruptly, presenting with mental confusion, staggering gait, and ocular abnormalities. Other physical and mental abnormalities are observed. In some patients, mild delirium occurs in which perceptual distortions and various types of hallucinations are reported. In a small percentage of patients, the delirium may escalate to frank delirium tremens, but when this occurs, it is always evanescent and usually not severe (Lishman, 1987).

Occasionally, Wernicke's encephalopathy may develop simultaneously with delirium tremens. In such cases, symptoms of both syndromes are identified and treated promptly. It is common medical practice to give thiamine and multivitamins to patients with delirium tremens or during alcohol detoxification treatment prophylactically because these patients are at high risk of developing Wernicke's encephalopathy.

As in delirium tremens, Wernicke's encephalopathy is considered an acute medical emergency. Patients should be treated in the hospital with various supportive measures. Thiamine and multivitamins are given intravenously or intramuscularly until a normal diet is resumed. Oral preparations may then be administered. Agitated patients may require appropriate sedation. When hallucinations occur, small doses of a high potency antispychotic medication are usually effective.

Korsakoff's Psychosis

It is generally agreed upon that Korsakoff's psychosis represents the residual and sometimes permanent defect that is precipitated initially by untreated Wernicke's encephalopathy. The syndrome is characterized by memory disturbances and confabulation. Significant personality deterioration and social impairment may occur. Despite the term "psychosis" associated with the entity, no traditional psychotic symptoms such as hallucinations or delusions are usually reported as part of Korsakoff's syndrome. In fact, DSM-III-R classifies this condition under "Alcohol Amnestic Disorder" (DSM-III-R, 1987).

DIAGNOSTIC PROBLEMS

The occurrence of hallucinatory symptoms in association with alcoholism raises a serious question that is often very difficult to answer: Are these hallucinations part of the alcoholic syndrome, or do they represent the symptoms of a separate psychiatric disorders? The clinical manifestations of visual and tactile hallucinations during delirium tremens are quite typical and can be recognized and diagnosed easily in most cases. However, the onset of auditory hallucinations—especially in states of clear consciousness, after the delirious state has subsided, as in the case of alcoholic hallucinosis—may confront the clinician with a difficult diagnostic dilemma. As mentioned earlier, auditory hallucinations of alcoholic hallucinosis may resemble to a great extent those of schizophrenia. The differential diagnosis becomes even more difficult when alcoholic hallucinosis is associated with delusions or inappropriate affect (DSM-III-R, 1987).

Several investigators have attempted to study the hallucinatory phenomena associated with alcoholism. Some questioned whether such an entity actually exists. Scott et al. (1969) supported the notion that alcoholic hallucinosis was a "waste basket" from the diagnostic point of view. They concluded that alcoholic hallucinosis was not a clinical entity, and that the syndrome was not a unitary condition, but rather the end result of various causal factors. Furthermore, they felt that many patients who are labeled with alcoholic hallucinosis syndrome may, in fact, suffer from other psychiatric disorders such as schizophrenia or manic depressive illness.

However, despite the controversy, clinical evidence and the literature acknowledge the existence of a group of patients with a history of heavy alcohol dependence who suffer from chronic hallucinatory syndrome that cannot be explained by other psychiatric conditions. In fact, it is likely that such patients are frequently misdiagnosed as chronic schizophrenics (Surawicz, 1980). Deiker and Chambers (1978) attempted to compare the structure and the content of hallucinations in alcohol withdrawal and "functional" psychosis. They reported that alcoholic patients experienced fewer auditory and gustatory hallucinations than the patients with "functional" psychoses. Furthermore, they indicated that alcoholics experience more "animal" content, whereas the "functional" psychotics reported more "human" content in visual and auditory hallucinations. Goodwin et al. (1971) concluded that hallucinations alone could not be used as a diagnostic tool to differentiate between alcoholic hallucinosis and other psychiatric conditions associated with hallucinations.

In spite of the difficulties involved in distinguishing alcoholic hallucinosis from schizophrenia, several clinical guidelines are available. The age of onset of alcohol hallucinosis is usually later in life, commonly between the ages of forty and sixty, and the first episode occurs typically after ten years or more of heavy drinking. Unlike schizophrenia, the clinical manifestations of alcohol hallucinosis often appear suddenly toward the end of an extended period of alcohol intoxication, as the alcohol blood level begins to drop. Alcoholic hallucinosis is often accompanied by anxiety and depression, and the affect is appropriate to the nature of the experience. Usually the patient is aware of the unreality of the hallucination and is disturbed by it. In addition, most patients with alcoholic hallucinosis have no delusions and show no evidence of a formal thought disorder. However, cognitive impairment and intellectual dysfunction may interfere significantly with their thinking process and communicating abilities. Although alcohol hallucinosis may take a chronic course and persist for years, most cases, unlike schizophrenia, resolve within weeks or months, and respond to lower doses of antipsychotics than is needed with schizophrenia. Finally it is important to evaluate the family history of the patient. Generally there is no evidence of a positive history of schizophrenia among alcoholic relatives. It is important to keep in mind that alcohol hallucinosis is a relatively rare condition, therefore, other causes of hallucinations need to be ruled out before a final diagnosis is made (Surawicz, 1980; DSM-III-R, 1987).

One of the most difficult situations that mental health professionals face is patients with what is known as "dual diagnoses," i.e., primary psychiatric disorder such as schizophrenia or bipolar disorder coupled with substance abuse or dependence. In addition to the treatment problems and limitations of resources available to such patients, it is extremely difficult to differentiate between symptoms presenting as part of the psychiatric condition and those arising because of the substance abuse or dependence disorder. A classic example of this dilemma is a patient with schizophrenia and alcohol dependence. Chronic auditory hallucinations may be due to either condition, or both. The differential diagnosis becomes more difficult when most other schizophrenic symptoms such as delusions and thought disorder subside while auditory hallucinations persist.

SUMMARY

Hallucinations associated with alcohol withdrawal syndrome (delirium tremens) usually consist of visual perceptions that are often vivid and complex. Tactile hallucinations are also common. These hallucinatory experiences are usually accompanied by changes in the vital signs and alteration in the level of consciousness.

Alcohol hallucinosis refers to a state of auditory hallucinations that develops after the resolution of the delirious state. Typically, the patient is alert and oriented, and is aware of the unreality of his or her perceptions. Some cases of alcohol hallucinosis can persist for months and even, in rare instances, for years.

Differential diagnosis is important but may be difficult, especially in the "dually diagnosed" population.

8 ═

Hallucinations in Organic Mental Disorders

Organic mental disorders refer to a group of syndromes characterized by various psychiatric and behavioral disturbances induced by physical factors that affect the brain directly or indirectly. Pathological processes such as bleeding, infection, trauma, or tumors may involve the brain itself or the surrounding structures leading to various physical and psychiatric manifestations. On the other hand, the brain may be affected indirectly by systemic conditions such as septicemia, uremia, and other metabolic and toxic conditions that can present with neurological and psychiatric symptoms. These symptoms include: agitation, disorientation, memory disturbances, personality changes, anxiety, depression, delusions, and hallucinations.

CLINICAL PRESENTATIONS OF HALLUCINATORY SYMPTOMS

Organic mental disorders frequently result in perceptual abnormalities. Patients with such conditions commonly experience fleeting and changeable misinterpretations and illusions. The visual modality is affected more often than any other. Strangers may be perceived as family members or vice versa. A nurse approaching the patient with a syringe may be seen by the patient as an enemy ready to attack with a knife. Auditory illusions may also occur in organic mental disorders. In such instances, the patient may perceive ordinary noises in the room as threats.

Pseudohallucinations, as well as true hallucinations, are fairly common in organic mental disorders. The most frequent form is in the visual modality. Typically visual hallucinations are simple and unformed. They often consist of flashes of light, circles, lines, stars, or colors. Less frequently, visual hallucinations become more formed and consist of people, animals, or events taking place in front of the patient. Lilliputian hallucinations may occur, where people or animals are seen reduced in size. These hallucinations seem to intensify at night, in darkened surroundings, or when the eyes are closed. Most patients fully accept these experiences as real and may participate and react accordingly, usually with fear and apprehension, but sometimes with interest or even amusement. Although such hallucinations are organic in nature, they are heavily influenced by the psychological and cultural background of the patient.

Tactile hallucinations are frequently found in organic brain disorders, especially in substance intoxication or withdrawal. Most often, patients experience small insects crawling over their skin. Other tactile perceptions such as feelings of vibration or sexual stimulation may occur. Some patients with organic psychosis may report having bodily sensations imposed on them from the outside, such as feeling the effect of certain external forces moving them or controlling their actions.

Auditory hallucinations are less frequent in organic mental disorders. When they occur, they are unformed and usually consist of hearing footsteps, hums, whistles, or similar sounds. More complex hallucinations, such as music or names, also occur. Formed auditory hallucinations consisting of sentences and conversations are reported less often in organic mental disorders, but they are not uncommon. Cummings (1988) reported that patients with organic psychosis may have Schneiderian first-rank symptoms in which the patient experiences auditory hallucinations that are very similar to those of schizophrenia. Formed auditory hallucinations are particularly reported in cases of alcoholic hallucinosis.

Olfactory and gustatory hallucinations are found in certain organic mental disorders, and they are particularly common in neurological disorders, especially in temporal lobe epilepsy and uncinate gyrus fits.

CLINICAL SYNDROMES

Delirium

The essential features of delirium include: reduced ability to maintain attention to external stimuli, disorganized thinking, incoherent speech, alteration in the level of consciousness, agitation, disorientation, memory disturbances, illusions, and hallucinations. Other psychiatric symptoms may also occur. They include anxiety, fear, irritability, depression, euphoria, apathy, and delusional thinking. Neurological and physical signs and symptoms may be present, depending on the etiology of the delirious state.

Causes of delirium include: systemic infections, metabolic disorders such as hypoxia, hypercarbia, hypoglycemia, electrolyte imbalance, hepatic or renal failure, thiamine deficiency, psychoactive substance intoxication and withdrawal, and postoperative states. Delirium may also occur following head trauma, hypertensive encephalopathy, or seizures. Certain focal lesions within the right parietal lobe or the lower aspect of the occipital lobe may manifest with delirious states as well (DSM-III-R, 1987).

Delirium seems to occur more frequently among children and the elderly.

In the case of children, it is believed that the immature brain, probably due to incomplete myelination of brain cells, increases the vulnerability of the brain to delirious states. Similarly, in the case of the elderly, it appears that the degeneration process of brain cells along with the atherosclerotic changes in cerebral blood vessels render the aging brain susceptible to the development of delirium. In addition, preexisting brain damage, such as that produced by strokes, seems to increase the chances of developing delirious states.

Perceptual disturbances are very common in delirium. Visual and auditory illusions are frequent. Hallucinations are mostly of the visual type, but as mentioned earlier, auditory, tactile, gustatory, and olfactory hallucinations can also occur. Most hallucinatory experiences are simple and unformed, however, complex visual and auditory hallucinations may develop. Patients may harm themselves or others while attempting to flee frightening hallucinations.

Most delirious states subside within a short period of time, about one week. In rare cases, the symptoms may last longer, depending on the persistence of the organic condition. In all cases, early diagnosis and prompt treatment of the underlying organic cause will determine the speed of recovery and the final outcome.

ICU Psychosis and Postcardiotomy Delirium

Patients who are placed in the intensive care unit due to critical medical illness or following major surgical procedures may occasionally develop organic psychotic states. Visual hallucinations are frequent in such states. Other forms of hallucination may also occur. When psychotic states follow heart surgery, it is referred to as postcardiotomy delirium. Kornfeld et al. (1978) reported that such psychotic states develop in approximately 10–20 percent of patients undergoing heart surgery. Eisendrath et al. (1983) reported the occurrence of visual hallucinations in association with disorientation in patients with Guillian-Barre syndrome, especially in those patients who are bound to ventilators in the intensive care unit.

Hallucinations experienced in the intensive care unit may be precipitated by multiple causes. However, lack of sleep and sensory deprivation play a significant role.

Hallucinations Associated with AIDS

It is known that Acquired Immune Deficiency Syndrome (AIDS) involves the central nervous system. Navia et al. (1986) reported that seven percent of AIDS patients in their study presented with an organic psychosis as the initial manifestation of the illness, and 16 percent exhibited psychotic symptoms later on during the course of the disease. Hallucinatory symptoms have been reported as part of the early manifestation of AIDS dementia which occurs due to the direct CNS involvement with the AIDS virus. In addition, hallucinations may develop in the course of delirious states resulting from secondary infections and other medical complications associated with AIDS (Navia & Price, 1986).

Hallucinations Associated with Encephalitis

Central nervous system infections, such as herpes encephalitis and Jakob-Creutzfeld disease, may produce an organic psychosis (Cummings, 1988). Various forms of meningitis and encephalitis have been implicated in some cases of hallucinations associated with delirium (Lewis, 1982). In a self report, Mize (1980) described experiencing visual hallucinations following viral encephalitis. Tertiary syphilis involving the CNS, a condition formerly known as General Paralysis of the Insane, was described as manifesting with hallucinations in addition to other psychological and neurological symptoms (Lishman, 1987).

Metabolic and Toxic Encephalopathies

Several metabolic and toxic pathological conditions may lead to systemic manifestations and affect the central nervous system in a generalized way. Encephalopathy refers to the global involvement of the brain with a pathological process that may lead to physical, neurological, and psychiatric manifestations. Most often encephalopathy presents as a delirium with all of its psychological and behavioral symptoms. Hallucinatory symptoms occur in encephalopathy, and as in delirium, they are mainly of the visual modality.

Various endocrine disorders, such as adrenocortical hypofunction, thyroid disorders, parathyroid disorders, and Vitamin D intoxication can result in several psychiatric symptoms, including hallucinations (Lewis, 1982; Hall, 1983). Nutritional deficiency states, such as starvation, beriberi, pellagra, and rare cases of hypoglycemia have been reported to produce hallucinatory symptoms (Simonds, 1986). Electrolyte and mineral disturbances may cause organic psychotic states. Copper and zinc deficiencies (Hansen et al., 1983) and hypomagnesemia (Lewis, 1982) have been noted to manifeset with hallucinatory symptoms in certain patients.

Acute liver failure due to viral hepatitis or Wilson's disease may result in hepatic encephalopathy, which may manifest with organic psychotic symptoms, including hallucinations (Lishman, 1987). Similarly, acute or end-stage renal failure may cause uremic encephalopathy with organic psychosis and hallucinations. Porphyria may manifest with a similar clinical picture as well (Weiner, 1961).

Intoxication with various chemical agents and poisons may produce toxic encephalopathies. Toxic levels of carbon dioxide, mercury, and bromide can lead to delirious states with hallucinations (Shader, 1972; Maghazaji, 1974). Visual hallucinations of "nets" were reported as part of the organic reaction seen in bromide intoxication when this preparation was in common use (Lishman, 1987).

Hallucinations Associated with Dementias

The essential features of dementia include: memory disturbance, gradual loss of abstract thinking, impaired judgment, and personality changes. Dementia is found predominantly in the elderly, but it may occur at any age. Common causes of dementia include primary degenerative dementia (Alzheimer's disease) and multi-infarct dementia. Several other metabolic, infectious, and neurological conditions may lead to various forms of dementia (DSM-III-R, 1987).

Psychotic symptoms are not uncommon in dementia. Cummings (1988) found that patients with dementia syndromes exhibited both simple unstructured delusions, as well as complex highly structured delusional beliefs. Visual, tactile, and auditory hallucinations have been reported in patients with Alzheimer's disease and multi-infarct dementia. Sulkava (1982) indicated that hallucinations are common in the middle and later stages of Alzheimer's disease. However, Crystal et al. (1988) reported on a patient with Alzheimer's disease who presented with visual hallucinations as the first symptom of the disease. Cummings et al. (1987) noted that auditory hallucinations were rare among psychotic patients with Alzheimer's disease and multi-infarct dementia. Gilchrist and Kalucy (1983) reported the occurrence of musical hallucinations in an elderly patient in association with worsening of dementia symptoms. They added that visual and tactile hallucinations also developed in the absence of any delirious symptoms. They suggested that a global degenerative process with possible involvement of the temporal cortical association area may be a contributory mechanism to those hallucinations.

Hallucinations in Other Organic Conditions

Hallucinatory symptoms have been reported among patients with cardiac and respiratory insufficiencies (Weiner, 1961). Decreased cerebral blood flow and reduced oxygenation of the brain may be responsible in such conditions. Allen and Agus (1968) reported cases of hallucinations induced by hyperventilation in teenagers. They speculated that vasoconstriction of cerebral blood vessels may precipitate those experiences. Systemic Lupus Erythematosis with central nervous system involvement may present with visual hallucinations and other psychiatric symptoms (Silber et al., 1984). Some patients with temporal arteritis have been reported to have hallucinations as well (Asaad & Shapiro, 1986).

Organic Hallucinosis

Hallucinosis refers to hallucinatory symptoms that occur in clear states of consciousness, and generally in the absence of other psychotic symptoms such as delusions or thought disorder. These hallucinations are usually persistent or recurrent and can be attributed to certain specific organic factors. Etiologic factors include: prolonged use of alcohol, use of hallucinogens, blindness, deafness, seizure foci in the temporal and occipital lobes, and prolonged sensory deprivation. Hallucinations may involve any sensory modality, but they are most commonly visual or auditory. They can vary from simple and unformed to extremely complex and well organized hallucinations. Most patients recognize the unreality of the hallucinations and may be disturbed by them, however, some individuals may believe in the reality of their experiences with delusional certainty (Kaplan & Sadock, 1985).

Hallucinations Induced by Alcohol and Other Psycho-Active Substances

Hallucinations may occur as a result of prolonged alcohol abuse and withdrawal. These hallucinations are discussed in detail in Chapter 7. Hallucinations induced by hallucinogenic drugs and related substances are discussed in Chapter 9.

Hallucinations as Side Effect of Medications

Hallucinations as well as other psychotic symptoms may develop as side effects to various medications and pharmacological agents. These hallucinations are discussed in Chapter 10.

Hallucinations Associated with Neurological Disorders

Various types of hallucinations may occur in several neurological conditions. They are discussed in Chapter 11.

Hallucinations Associated with Ear and Eye Diseases

Hallucinatory phenomena have been reported in patients with deafness or blindness. These hallucinations are discussed in Chapter 12.

DIFFERENTIAL DIAGNOSIS

Although most hallucinatory symptoms associated with organic states are in the visual modality, and of the simple unformed nature, some hallucinations may be identical to those of idiopathic or "functional" psychotic states. In fact, Goodwin et al. (1971) found that hallucinatory symptoms were nonspecific and could not be used alone to differentiate between one condition and another. Nevertheless, hallucinations in organic psychotic conditions have common clinical characteristics that may distinguish them from those caused by other conditions. The age of onset may be at any age, but usually it is later in life. The clinical manifestations are variable, and sometimes may be accompanied by delirium or dementia. The patient generally has a normal premorbid personality and often has no history of psychiatric illness. Family history often provides further clinical evidence in support of one diagnosis or another. Finally, a careful history and a meticulous physical examination with the identification of neurological and medical problems are essential in reaching a final diagnosis (Cummings, 1988).

TREATMENT OF ORGANICALLY INDUCED HALLUCINATIONS

It is extremely important to keep in mind that the focus of the treatment should be on the underlying organic condition that has led to the hallucinatory symptoms. However, organic psychosis responds very well to antipsychotic medications, which are very helpful in controlling the patient's agitation and unpredictable behavior. Psychiatrists should use small doses of high potency neuroleptic medications, as low potency neuroleptics are more likely to cause hypotensive or anticholinergic reactions that may exacerbate the organic condition. This is of particular importance in elderly patients who must be evaluated carefully for the potentially harmful side effects of medications, such as hypotensive episodes that may lead to falls with possible hip fracture or other injuries. In most patients, the doses needed to control the psychotic symptoms are much lower than those needed for "functional" psychotic states such as schizophrenia or mania. The dosage should be titrated downwards as the symptoms are brought under control. In addition it is not required that most patients be kept on the antipsychotic medication beyond a few days after the hallucinatory symptoms have stopped. It is generally recommended that such medications be discontinued gradually over several days. Cummings (1988) warned that patients with underlying extrapyramidal diseases, such as Parkinson's disease, may have their movement disorder exacerbated by neuroleptic agents and may be more prone to the development of Tardive Dyskinesia. He recommended that neuroleptic medications should be used sparingly if at all in such circumstances.

Benzodiazepines have also been shown to be helpful in the treatment of hallucinatory symptoms in certain conditions (Asaad & Shapiro, 1986). Such agents may be effective in reducing the patient's fear and anxiety as well. Treatment of hallucinations with other medications or methods is discussed in detail in Chapter 17.

SUMMARY

Hallucinations that occur in the course of an organic mental disorder usually consist of simple visual perceptions, though more complex visual hallucinations can also occur. Less frequently, auditory and tactile hallucinations may be reported. Olfactory and gustatory hallucinations usually develop in association with seizure disorders. The underlying etiology should be identified and treated accordingly. However, a small dose of a high potency antipsychotic agent is usually effective in alleviating the hallucinatory symptoms.

9

Hallucinogenic Drugs and Other Psychoactive Substances

Most drugs have been known and used for various purposes throughout recorded history. However, the sharp rise in the recreational use of drugs is a relatively recent phenomenon that started during the nineteenth century, and has continued to the present time. The recent explosion in drug abuse, especially of cocaine, has created a national and an international dilemma, and has focused the attention on the medical aspects and social implications of long-term use of such agents.

BIOLOGICAL CONSIDERATIONS

Hallucinogens and other psychoactive substances affect the CNS and produce a variety of profound effects on behavior, mood, thought, and perception. The extensive research in the 50s and 60s on hallucinogens, and in the past two decades on various drugs has led to a significant body of knowledge concerning the behavioral and physiological effects of these agents.

Winters (1975) proposed that hallucinogens produce their effects by shifting the electrical activity of the CNS toward an arousal pattern and by impairing information input at the same time. West (1975) suggested that the hallucinogenic characteristics of LSD may be due to its effect as a "sensory poison" and as a cortical arouser. It is currently believed that hallucinogens act by altering various neurotransmitters in the brain such as serotonin and dopamine (Fischman, 1983).

Wooley and Shaw (1954) noted the structural similarity between LSD and serotonin molecules and postulated that a blockade of central serotonin receptors might account for the psychotic symptoms produced by LSD. Other researchers found later that LSD specifically inhibits unit activity of dorsal raphe neurons. In fact, it was concluded that every major member of the

52

class of hallucinogenic drugs or agents that can cause hallucinatory experiences was uniquely capable of exerting a pronounced inhibitory effect on the serotonin-containing neurons of the dorsal raphe nucleus. However, other psycho-active drugs such as opiates, atropine, and tetrahydrocannabinol (THC) did not produce such effects (Fischman, 1983).

Amphetamine was found to act through increasing dopaminergic activity, thus producing paranoid and hallucinatory symptoms (Meltzer & Stahl, 1976). Trulson and Jacobs (1979b) later demonstrated that amphetamine, in addition to its effect on dopamine, when administered for a long time, results in a significant decrease in serotonin and 5-HIAA concentrations in the brain. Although clinical experience with human ingestion of amphetamines indicates that hallucinations develop after a prolonged administration of high doses of the drug, there are some reports of hallucinations developing after short periods of ingestion, perhaps as short as several days and at low doses. Young (1981) suggested that it is possible that amphetamines may also act by direct effect on the noradrenergic neurons in the lateral geniculate nucleus.

The effect of hallucinogens on serotonin metabolism was at one time believed to take place largely at the presynaptic sites. However, it has been shown recently that hallucinogenic drugs produce the behavioral and perceptual changes by acting on the postsynaptic serotonergic neurons. Heym et al. (1984) administered mianserin (a serotonin antagonist that acts mainly at the postsynaptic 5-HT2 receptor sites) to cats 30 minutes before giving the hallucinogens. They found that the behavioral effects of the hallucinogens were blocked by mianserin, whereas the presynaptic effect of the hallucinogen, namely, decreased firing of the 5-HT neurons, was unaffected.

Domino and Ruffing (1982) suggested that opioid receptors play a role in the behavioral response to hallucinogens. They argued that opioid antagonists can potentiate the behavioral effect of both DMT and LSD.

Brandys and Yehuda (1983) suggested that LSD and other hallucinogens act as dopamine agonists and that they have an inhibitory effect on the monoamine oxidase enzymes. Low platelet MAO activity has been implicated in the mechanism of hallucinatory phenomena.

It has been suggested (Wells, 1985) that hallucinogenic drugs stimulate neurons in the temporal lobe and in the limbic system leading to electrophysiological and neurochemical reactions that result in hallucinatory experiences. Repeated use of hallucinogens is likely to cause abnormal neuronal activity deep within the brain structures and may even result in persistent anatomical changes as well. Eventually these changes may predispose the neurons in the temporal lobe and the limbic system structures to produce spontaneous paroxysmal discharges in the absence of hallucinatory drug effect. Such recurrent neuronal activity may account for the persistence of hallucinatory symptoms in certain individuals long after they have stopped using drugs. These changes in neuronal activity appear to be reversible, at least up to a certain point, if stimulation with hallucinogens is discontinued.

However, if hallucinogens are abused for a long time, permanent changes may result, leading to chronic hallucinations or recurrent hallucinatory experiences known as "flashbacks" (Wells, 1985). Fischer (1971) proposed that flashbacks resulted from inducing a certain level of arousal that had prevailed during the initial hallucinatory experience.

CLINICAL FEATURES

Hallucinations induced by drugs are essentially similar to those encountered in organic psychotic states. They are predominantly visual, with vivid colors and images. Typically the hallucinatory experience starts with unformed visual sensations with alterations of color, size, shape, and movement. The images are usually abstract, such as lines, stars, and flashes of light. Gradually more formed visual hallucinations develop with images of people, objects, or events. These hallucinations are more readily seen with the eyes closed or in darkened surroundings.

Auditory hallucinations have been reported in cases of drug-induced psychosis as well. When they occur, they are usually unformed and are experienced as indistinct noises. However, these hallucinations can become more formed and be heard as music or even voices which may resemble to a great extent schizophrenic hallucinations.

Tactile hallucinations (also known as haptic hallucinations) are experienced during drug intoxications. Most often individuals feel small insects crawling up their skin. (This condition is known as formication.)

Some patients who are under the influence of psychedelic drugs experience "synesthetic hallucinations," wherein the individual may perceive colorful visual hallucinations after hearing a loud noise, or may have auditory hallucinations in response to a bright light. It has been suggested that this phenomenon occurs because of drug-induced cortical hypersensitivity, which allows a strong stimulus in one area to trigger other areas of the cortex (Asaad & Shapiro, 1986).

In some individuals who chronically abuse hallucinogenic drugs, episodic recurrences of portions of prior hallucinatory experiences may occur. These hallucinations are known as "flashbacks." Flashbacks are spontaneous recurrences of illusions and visual hallucinations that happen during a drug-free state similar to those experienced during the active stage of drug administration. Flashbacks can occur months or even years after initial drug use (Horowitz, 1969). After chronic and heavy hallucinogen abuse, some patients develop persistent hallucinatory psychoses. The clinical picture in such cases may be indistinguishable from chronic schizophrenia, especially when patients develop thought disorder as well (Wells, 1985).

Most patients are usually aware of the unreality of the experiences, however, some individuals believe these hallucinations with delusional certainty. Unlike schizophrenic patients, these individuals often are eager to tell others of the vivid, intense, and continuous nature of their hallucinatory experiences. Some patients may be visibly distressed by these hallucinations and may shout and rail against their perceptions. Others may be calm and amused by them. It is important to keep in mind that a certain drug may not produce the same hallucinatory effect every time. Effects may vary according to the person, dose, mood, social setting, and physical condition. On the other hand, the same hallucinatory experience may be induced by a wide variety of drugs. In all cases, the nature and the content of the hallucinatory experience is greatly influenced by the individual's psychological background (Asaad & Shapiro, 1986).

In addition to hallucinatory symptoms, drugs tend to produce a wide variety of other psychiatric and physical symptoms. Paranoid delusions, anxiety, and affective changes are common. Tachycardia, sweating, pupillary dilation, tremor, and incoordination occur with some drugs. Clinical presentation may vary depending on the type of drug used. These conditions are described below.

Hallucinogens

Hallucinogenic drugs are substances that produce perceptual distortion when administered in low doses that are insufficient to produce a toxic delirious condition. Hallucinogens are also known as "psychedelic" (mind-realizing) drugs, which refers to their seeming ability to expand perceptual and experiential horizons (West, 1975). There are many hallucinogenic drugs, some natural and some synthetic. The best known drugs include lysergic acid diethylamide (LSD), mescaline, and psilocybin. Other hallucinogens include; harmine, harmaline, ibogaine, dimethyltryptamine (DMT), diethyltryptamine (DET), dipropyltryptamine (DPT), 3,4-methylenedioxyamphetamine (MDA), and 2,5-dimethoxy-4-methylamphetamine (DOM, also known as STP). Only LSD and to some extent MDA are now available in any quantity on the illicit market (Grinspoon & Bakalar, 1985).

LSD produces profound alterations in perception, mood, and thinking. Perceptions usually become brilliant and intense. All of the senses are enhanced and the individual is usually more attentive to details. Colors and textures seem richer. Visual distortions and pseudohallucinations are common. True visual hallucinations also occur. Auditory and tactile hallucinations are rarely present. Synesthesia is particularly common. Changes in body image and alterations in the perception of time and space also occur. Depersonalization and derealization may develop. Physical symptoms include pupillary dilation, tachycardia, sweating, palpitations, blurring of vision, tremor, and incoordination (DSM-III-R, 1987).

The onset of hallucinatory symptoms is usually within one hour of drug ingestion, and the condition lasts approximately six hours, but in some instances it may last as long as three days. It is not unusual for severe emotional disturbance in the form of severe panic reaction or psychotic state to accompany LSD intoxication. This adverse effect has been described by users as a "bad trip" (Walker & Cavenar, 1983).

Flashbacks occur frequently after the ingestion of LSD in a drug-free state. Probably about 25 percent of all psychedelic drug users have experienced some form of flashback. Flashbacks usually are mild and they decrease quickly in number and intensity with time. Such episodes are most likely to occur under stress. Fatigue, drunkenness, marijuana intoxication, or severe illness may precipitate flashbacks (Grinspoon & Bakalar, 1985).

Recreational use of hallucinogenic drugs has declined lately and cocaine and marijuana are the prevalent drugs of choice.

Phencyclidine (PCP)

Phencyclidine is a white crystal that can be quite easily manufactured and is known on the street as "Angel Dust" or "Crystal." PCP may be taken by mouth, intravenously, or snorted. Chronic users prefer to smoke it. There are about 30 chemical analogues of PCP. Ketamine, a short acting anesthetic, is a related drug with psychoactive properties, similar to those of phencyclidine.

Physical symptoms begin five minutes after the drug is smoked or taken intravenously. They include nystagmus, elevated blood pressure, diminished responsiveness to pain, ataxia, dysarthria, and diaphoresis (Walker & Cavenar, 1983). Psychiatric symptoms begin with euphoria, bodily warmth, tingling, peaceful floating sensations, and depersonalization. Later, striking alterations in body image, distortions of space and time perception, synesthesia, auditory or visual hallucinations, and delusions develop. Severe anxiety, agitation, assaultiveness, or bizarre behavior sometimes occur. Intoxication generally lasts three to six hours, and most patients will completely recover within a day or two. However, some patients will remain psychotic for as long as two weeks (Grinspoon & Bakalar, 1985).

Marijuana

Marijuana is prepared from the hemp plant, cannabis sativa. Preparations obtained from various species or ecotypes are known as cannabinols. These drugs are known as hashish, bhang, kif, marijuana, pot, and various other names. The active constituents of the plant are various isomers of tetrahydrocannabinol (THC). THC has been known to produce an LSD-like reaction in higher doses, clearly making it a hallucinogenic drug (West, 1975). The drug can be taken as a drink or in foods, but most frequently it is smoked either in a pipe or in a cigarette, referred to as a joint (Grinspoon, 1977).

Intoxication occurs almost immediately after smoking marijuana, peaks within a half hour and usually lasts about three hours. Symptoms include euphoria, anxiety, paranoia, sensation of slowed time, impaired judgment, and social withdrawal. Inappropriate laughter, panic attacks, and dysphoric mood may be experienced. Individuals may feel that they are dying or losing their mind. When very high blood levels are reached, perceptual abnormalities start to develop. Distortions of body parts, spatial and temporal distortions, depersonalization, derealization, increased sensitivity to sound, synesthesia, and true hallucinations may be experienced. Physical symptoms include conjunctival injection, tachycardia, increased appetite, and a dry mouth. There are some indications of tolerance and a mild withdrawal effect after frequent use of high doses, but there is no clinical evidence that withdrawal symptoms lead to any significant addictive problem among chronic users (DSM-III-R, 1987).

Cocaine

Cocaine sold on the street varies greatly in purity. It is usually cut with sugar, procaine, or other substances. Cocaine is administered mainly by snuffing (snorting), subcutaneous or intravenous injection, or freebasing (smoked in a pipe or cigarette). The effect of cocaine is almost instant, with initial euphoria and sense of well-being. Grandiosity, hypervigilance, agitation, and impaired judgment may occur. Physical symptoms include tachycardia, pupillary dilation, elevated blood pressure, perspiration or chills, and nausea and vomiting. If the intoxication is severe, confusion, rambling, anxiety, and apprehension are likely to be present. Patients may experience paranoid ideations and hallucinations. Most often individuals experience tactile hallucinations; a sensation of insects crawling up the skin (formication). Visual hallucinations may occur in which patients report seeing small insects. Less frequently, auditory hallucinations are experienced as ringing in the ears, or hearing one's name called (DSM-III-R, 1987; Khantzian, 1983).

Siegel (1978) reported that cocaine can produce hallucinatory symptoms of all modalities. He noted that the most frequent type of hallucination was visual hallucinations, followed by tactile hallucinations, and then by olfactory hallucinations. Auditory and gustatory types were least common. Siegel (1978) pointed out the similarity of cocaine hallucinations to "entoptic phenomena" (that arise from the visualization of certain structures within the eye through the appropriate arrangement of incident light). He also noted that cocaine hallucinations were very similar to migraine hallucinations. He proposed that such similarity suggests a common mechanism of action based on central nervous system excitation and arousal.

After the immediate psychoactive effects of high doses of cocaine have subsided, they are replaced by unpleasant rebound effects which make up what is known as the "crash"; including a dysphoric mood, a craving for cocaine, anxiety, tremulousness, irritability, and feeling of fatigue and depression. When these symptoms extend beyond 24 hours, the condition is referred to as cocaine withdrawal. Cocaine is now believed to be highly addictive, and the administration of large doses may result in syncope, chest pain, seizures, or even death due to cardiac arrhythmias or respiratory paralysis (DSM-III-R, 1987).

Amphetamines

Amphetamine and similarly acting sympathomimetic substances such as methylphenidate (Ritalin) lead to several psychiatric and physical manifestations. Behavioral and psychiatric symptoms include: agitation, dysphoria, insomnia, irritability, hostility, tension, anxiety, paranoid ideation, and visual, tactile, and auditory hallucinations. Physical symptoms include tachycardia, pupillary dilation, elevated blood pressure, perspiration or chills, and nausea and vomiting (Ellinwood et al., 1973; DSM-III-R, 1987). Amphetamine abuse may lead to intoxication, delirium, or delusions and may be indistinguishable from cocaine intoxication. Delusions and hallucinations are always transient in cocaine intoxication; whereas, delusions and hallucinations of amphetamine abuse may persist beyond the time of direct substance effect (Walker & Cavenar, 1983).

Inhalants and Volatile Solvents

Varnish remover, gasoline, lighter fluid, airplane glue, rubber cement, cleaning fluid, and aerosols such as spray paints are among the substances in this category. The active ingredients that produce addictive behavior include toluene, acetone, benzene, and halogenated hydrocarbons. Inhalants are central nervous system depressants that lead to euphoria, excitement, a floating sensation, dizziness, slurred speech, ataxia, and a sense of heightened power. Other features include belligerence, assaultiveness, and impaired judgment. The symptoms resemble those of alcohol and sedative intoxications (Grinspoon & Bakalar, 1985).

Chronic solvent abuse may lead to hallucinatory symptoms. Channer and Stanley (1983) reported a case of a 16-year-old boy who experienced persistent visual hallucinations from glue sniffing and who exhibited diffusely abnormal EEG and delayed visually evoked responses to checkerboard pattern reversal (VERS).

Benzodiazepines

Benzodiazepines have significant anxiolytic and sedative properties. Their effect is very similar to that of alcohol. Benzodiazepines may produce hallucinatory symptoms as part of their adverse effects. Viscott (1968) reported hallucinatory symptoms induced by chlordiazepoxide (Librium). This effect has been considered by some to be a manifestation of the excitement phase of sedation. Recent reports have implicated triazolam (Halcion) in causing visual hallucinations in some individuals.

Hallucinations seem to be more common as part of the withdrawal syndrome from benzodiazepines and barbiturates. These withdrawal symptoms are very similar to alcohol withdrawal symptoms (delirium tremens). Hallucinations induced by sedative-hypnotic drug intoxication and withdrawal are discussed in Chapter 10.

Methaqualone

Methaqualone (Quaalude) is a nonbarbiturate sedative-hypnotic. Overdose on methaqualone may produce delirious states that may include hallucinatory symptoms. In addition, withdrawal from the drug may precipitate hallucinations and nightmares (Grinspoon & Bakalar, 1985).

Opioids

Narcotics have been reported to produce hallucinatory symptoms (Jarvik, 1970). Hallucinations induced by opioid analgesics such as morphine, when used for the management of pain in certain patients, are discussed in Chapter 10.

TREATMENT

Hallucinations along with the rest of the psychotic syndrome are managed essentially as an organic psychotic state. It is believed that the nature and the extent of the psychotic reaction may vary from one person to another, depending on the person's biological vulnerability and environmental circumstances. In addition, patients with preexisting psychiatric conditions may have their psychiatric symptoms exacerbated as a result of the drug administration.

Hallucinations and other psychotic symptoms induced by drugs may be controlled effectively by benzodiazepines. However, in certain patients the use of antipsychotic medications may be necessary. As in organic psychosis, these symptoms respond well to small doses of a high potency antipsychotic medication such as haloperidol. Treatment of amphetamine and PCP psychosis may require ammonium chloride or ascorbic acid to acidify the urine in order to facilitate the elimination of the drug.

Khantzian (1983) reported that an extreme case of cocaine withdrawal responded very well to methylphenidate (Ritalin).

Chronic persistent hallucinations precipitated by repeated heavy hallucinogen abuse may be very resistant to treatment with antipsychotic medications. It has been suggested that anticonvulsant medications may be effective in some patients in whom neuroleptics have failed (Wells, 1985).

Other treatment modalities are discussed in Chapter 17.

SUMMARY

Various types of perceptual distortions, illusions, and hallucinations can be induced by hallucinogenic drugs and other psychoactive substances. Visual hallucinations occur more frequently than other types and seem to intensify with the eyes closed or in darkened surroundings. Hallucinatory reactions induced by a certain drug may vary depending on the person, dose, mood, and physical setting. Furthermore, the same hallucinatory experience may be induced by a wide variety of drugs. These hallucinations respond reasonably well to treatment with benzodiazepines, and antipsychotic medications.

10 ≡

Hallucinations Induced by Pharmacological Agents

Several pharmacological agents commonly used in clinical practice are capable of producing significant effects on the Central Nervous System leading to alterations of cognition, behavior, perception, affect, memory, thinking, and sleep patterns. The effect of these pharmacological agents may vary depending on the dose, the age of the patient, the underlying physical and psychiatric conditions, and several other biological and environmental factors.

The psychiatric symptoms induced by medications are usually similar to those encountered in organic mental disorders. Most often, the patient presents with delirium that may involve disorientation, alteration of level of consciousness, hallucinations, and delusions. Neurological and physical signs may be present. Occasionally, psychiatric symptoms such as hallucinations and paranoid delusions may develop in the absence of delirium.

As in other organic psychotic states, perceptual disturbances that occur as a side effect of medications usually involve the visual modality, leading to visual illusions, pseudohallucinations, and true hallucinations. Auditory, tactile, olfactory, and gustatory hallucinations can also occur. These hallucinations are usually simple and unformed, however, complex hallucinatory experiences may develop as well (Paulseth & Klawans, 1985).

PSYCHOTROPIC MEDICATIONS

Several psychotropic medications used for the treatment of various psychiatric disorders may affect the brain adversely and cause behavioral, cognitive, and perceptual disturbances.

Antidepressant Medications

The ability of tricyclic and tetracyclic antidepressants to block the reuptake of serotonin, norepinephrine, or dopamine by presynaptic terminals seems to be responsible for the production of various psychiatric and behavioral adverse effects of these medications. In addition, most antidepressants have prominent anticholinergic properties that may add to the toxic confusional state that often presents as an anticholinergic psychosis (Paulseth & Klawans, 1985).

Antidepressant medications have been reported to precipitate manic episodes in some patients with bipolar disorder when given during the depressive episode of the illness. Furthermore, antidepressants can activate schizophrenic symptoms in patients with preexisting disease.

Hallucinations, especially of the visual modality, have been reported as a side effect of various antidepressant medications. Hemmingsen and Rafaelsen (1980) reported the occurrence of hypnagogic and hypnopompic hallucinations among patients treated with amitriptyline. A recent report by Rundell and Murray (1988) noted that visual hallucinations may occur on a low dose of amitriptyline. Norman et al. (1982) described the occurrence of visual hallucinations in response to increased plasma concentration of doxepin and its metabolite. Barnes (1982) reported a case of an 87-year-old depressed patient who developed manic symptoms and visual hallucinations in response to treatment with amoxapine hydrochloride at 100 mgs per day. Damlouji and Ferguson (1984) implicated trazodone in producing delirium, including hallucinations and cognitive changes in patients with major depression associated with bulimia. Albala et al. (1983) reported two cases of hypnopompic hallucinations induced by maprotiline. Psychotic symptoms including hallucinations and delusions were reported among patients during clinical trials with the new antidepressant bupropion (Johnston et al., 1986). In addition, imipramine hydrochloride, a widely used tricyclic antidepressant, was reported to cause hallucinatory symptoms as well (Cummings & Miller, 1987).

MAO inhibitors have been noted by several clinicians to cause mania, to convert retarded depression into an agitated depression but rarely to cause a confusional state with hallucinations (Paulseth & Klawans, 1985; Cummings & Miller, 1987).

Benzodiazepines

The major effect of benzodiazepines on CNS involves the potentiation of gamma aminobutyric acid (GABA) system. They have significant sedative, anxiolytic and muscle relaxant effects. Unwanted side effects of benzodiazepines include confusion, excitement, agitation, hallucinations, and nightmares. Exacerbation of depression and psychosis have also been reported (Paulseth & Klawans, 1985; Viscott, 1968). Minichetti and Milles (1982) reported the occurrence of hallucinations and delirium as a result of intravenous diazepam administration. Hallucinations have also occurred in children after the oral administration of lorazepam (Van-den-Berg, 1986). In addition, several clinical reports have implicated the hypnotic agent triazolam (Halcion) as responsible for visual hallucinations and nightmares in some individuals.

Withdrawal from benzodiazepines resembles to a great extent alcohol withdrawal syndrome and may present with delirious states and hallucinatory experiences. Chandora (1980) reported a case of delayed diazepam withdrawal syndrome that included auditory and visual hallucinations, and seizures. Noyes et al. (1988) indicated that withdrawal syndrome from benzodiazepines causes depersonalization and heightened perception, including increased sensitivity to stimulation of various sensory modalities. They added that patients may experience perceptual distortions involving visual hallucinations and misperceptions of movements.

Lithium

Lithium has proven efficacy in acute mania, helps in some cases of depression, and prevents mood swings in bipolar patients. Psychiatric manifestations of lithium toxicity may include acute confusional state with disorientation, memory loss, thought disorder, and lability of mood. Patients with preexisting schizophrenia or brain damage seem to be more prone to develop this side effect (Paulseth & Klawans, 1985).

Hallucinations have occurred as an adverse effect of Lithium therapy. Sandyk and Gillman (1985) reported increased visual hallucinations in response to lithium treatment. Such hallucination disappeared completely when the patient was given naloxon. They suggested that lithium induced hallucinations may be mediated by the indogenous opioid system. A recent report by Price et al. (1989) indicated that lithium treatment enhances serotoninergic function. The ability of lithium to induce hallucinations in certain individuals may be related to its effect on the serotonergic system.

CENTRAL STIMULANTS

Stimulants are characterized by sympathomimetic effects, and they appear to act through a release of norepinephrine and dopamine from presynaptic terminals. Stimulants include amphetamine, methylphenidate, and pemoline. In cases of acute toxicity, patients may develop delirium with psychiatric and behavioral disturbances, accompanied by sympathomimetic effects such as increased pulse, elevated blood pressure, diaphoresis, dilated pupils, and tremor. Tactile hallucinatons are particularly common (Ellinwood et al., 1973). When administered on a long-term basis, amphetamine can cause psychotic symptoms such as paranoid delusions, thought disorder, and hallucinations (Paulseth & Klawans, 1985).

Hallucinatory symptoms have been reported in up to 83 percent of chronic users of amphetamines (Paulseth & Klawans, 1985). Hawks et al. (1969) noted the predominance of visual and auditory types in such individuals. Lucas and Weiss (1971) reported the occurrence of similar hallucinatory syndromes as a result of methylphenidate use.

It is believed that psychotic reactions induced by these drugs may reflect excessive dopaminergic activity, perhaps within the limbic system or neocortex (Paulseth & Klawans, 1985).

ANTIPARKINSONIAN DRUGS, DOPAMINERGIC, AND ANTICHOLINERGIC AGENTS

Patients with Parkinson's disease who are treated with dopaminergic or anticholinergic drugs experience hallucinatory symptoms, mainly of the visual modality. Goetz et al. (1982) suggested that both the dopaminergic and the cholinergic systems are reciprocally active in the psychopathology of long-term, drug-induced hallucinatory states in this population.

Amantadine, a dopamine releasing agent, is known to induce various psychotic symptoms including hallucinations (Wilcox, 1985). Lisuride, another dopaminergic agent, when used in high doses for the treatment of Parkinson's disease, may produce visual hallucinations (Horowski, 1986). Other antiparkinsonian agents associated with hallucinations include levodopa, mesulergine, and pergolide mesylate (Cummings & Miller, 1987). Bromocriptine, a dopamine agonist, which is used for the treatment of certain endocrine disorders, neuroleptic malignant syndrome and Parkinson's disease, has been reported to produce hallucinatory symptoms (Harris, 1984).

Atropine and other anticholinergic drugs at high doses often precipitate toxic states associated with confusion, disorientation, depersonalization, paranoia, and hallucinations, particularly of the visual and tactile type (Greenblatt & Shader, 1973). Lilliputian hallucinations may occur. Physical symptoms include dry mucous membranes, mydriasis, blurred vision, photophobia, tachycardia, elevated temperature, urinary retention, constipation, and dry, warm skin. Benztropine and trihexyphenidyl, commonly used by psychiatrists in conjunction with antipsychotic medications to counteract extrapyramidal side effects, are among the anticholinergic agents that can cause hallucinations (Wilcox, 1983). Scopolamine was shown to increase auditory hallucinations in experimental subjects. Warburton et al. (1985) proposed that hallucinatory experiences precipitated by scopolamine may result from the impairment of information processing induced by the drug.

Anticholinergic toxicity may be produced by several other drugs that possess strong anticholinergic side effects. Examples include tricyclic antidepressants, antipsychotic medications, antiemetics, and antihistamines. Also, street drugs are often cut with the anticholinergic stramonium. Elderly patients seem to be especially vulnerable to anticholinergic toxic effects of anticholinergic preparations, even at low doses (Paulseth & Klawans, 1985). Over-the-counter sleep preparations may contain scopolamine. Therefore, these drugs are likely to induce anticholinergic hallucinatory reactions (Hooper et al., 1979).

Anticholinergic psychotic states respond well to physostigmine, although repeated injections are often necessary. However, such cholinergic agents may also induce central toxic states characterized by confusion and hallucinations. Other cholinergic agents that can produce toxic hallucinatory states include organophosphorus insecticides (Paulseth & Klawans, 1985).

ANTIHISTAMINES AND DECONGESTANTS

Antihistamines, when taken in large doses, are often responsible for the onset of hallucinations, especially in children. Hays et al. (1980) indicated that hallucinations can occur following a modest overdose of tripelennamine. Woodward and Baldassano (1988) reported that oral administration and topical application of diphenhydramine may produce visual hallucinations in children. Actifed (triprolidine and pseudoephedrine) was reported to cause visual hallucinations in some children after the recommended dose of the drug was taken. The hallucinatory symptoms lasted for one week to four months (Sankey et al., 1984). Dungal (1984) reported a case of a four-year-old girl who developed visual hallucinations following the administration of a decongestant-expectorant medication that contained chlorpheniramine maleate, phenylpropanolamine hydrochloride, and dextromethorphan hydrobromide.

ANALGESICS AND NARCOTICS

Narcotics have been reported to induce hallucinatory symptoms (Jarvik, 1970). Patients who receive morphine and other related preparations have experienced hallucinatory symptoms. Jellema (1987) reported a case of a 62-year-old patient with terminal cancer who was receiving sustained-release morphine infusion. The patient reported visual hallucinations of small insects as the dose was increased to 100 mgs. per day. When morphine was stopped, the hallucinations disappeared. Analgesia was then changed into methadone suppositories 60 mgs. per day. About 20 days after starting the methadone, the patient began to hallucinate again. The hallucinations disappeared over two days, without a change in treatment, which suggests an increased tolerance for methadone. Fogarty and Murray (1987) noted that hallucinatory symptoms do occur as part of the psychiatric presentation of meperidine toxicity.

Other narcotics have been implicated with similar reactions. Pentazocine (Talwin) has been reported on occasion to produce hallucinations (Miller, 1975). Buprenorphine, a newer narcotic analgesic with a much longer duration of action than morphine, and with less pronounced side effects than morphine, was reported to cause hallucinatory symptoms. Paraskevaides (1988) reported a case of a 50-year-old man with no previous history of mental illness who developed auditory hallucinations of voices instructing him to perform various jobs on the ward, half an hour after he received 200 mgs. of buprenorphine sublingually. Eventually, the patient threw himself out of the window in response to command hallucinations, which he described later as being perceived as real at the time of the experience.

ANTIINFLAMMATORY AGENTS

Several antiinflammatory agents have been implicated in the production of hallucinatory symptoms. Indomethacin is known to have high incidence of mild toxicity. It may cause headache, agitation, ataxia, depression, and hallucinations (Mills, 1974). Other antiinflammatory analgesic drugs such as salicylate and phenacetin have also been described to induce hallucinatory symptoms (Cummings & Miller, 1987). Allen (1985) reported a case of a 17-year-old patient with a history of arthritis and otosclerosis who developed a three-week history of hearing music that lasted all day unless there was another noise to interfere with it. She informed her physician that she had been taking 12 tablets of aspirin per day. Salicylate blood level was 36mg/100 ml (therapeutic range : 0–30). The music stopped in a few days after the patient reduced her aspirin intake to six tablets per day.

Corticosteroids can induce psychiatric symptoms. Most commonly, patients present with a hypomanic picture. Depression occurs less frequently. Other side effects include: depersonalization, labile affect, confusion, paranoia, mutism, and hallucinations (Paulseth & Klawans, 1985). Hallucinations are more likely to occur after changes in steroid dosage (Silber et al., 1984).

ANTICONVULSANT DRUGS

Anticonvulsant medications at toxic levels can produce a delirious state associated with ataxia, nystagmus, and altered level of consciousness. High phenytoin blood levels were correlated with dementia, depression, psychosis, myelopathy, and neuropathy in patients with vitamin B12 deficiency (Paulseth & Klawans, 1985). Cummings and Miller (1987) reported that visual hallucinations can occur with several anticonvulsant agents, including phenytoin, primidone, and phenobarbital. Simonds (1986) reported that high doses of anticonvulsant medications such as phenytoin can be associated with delirium, and auditory, tactile, and visual hallucinations. Van-Wieringen and Vrijlandt (1983) presented a case of a 21-year-old epileptic male who was treated with sodium valproate and ethosuximide. He was also on isoniazid. A rise and fall in ethosuximide blood levels paralleled the observation of psychotic episodes with delusions and hallucinations. They suggested that psychiatric symptoms may have occurred as a result of an interaction between ethosuximide and isoniazid.

ANAESTHETIC AGENTS

Hallucinations have been reported by patients who underwent anaesthesia (Lloyd, 1987). Nitrous oxide can cause hyperacusis, excitement, and delirium, especially if oxygen supply is limited (Frost, 1985). It has also been reported to induce hallucinatory symptoms in certain patients (Bennett, 1980).

Ketamine hydrochloride was reported to cause visual hallucinations (Cummings & Miller, 1987). Cunningham and McKinney (1983) suggested that ketamine produces a dissociation between the limbic system and the thalamocortical pathways. They reported that visual hallucinations associated with ketamine anesthesia usually involve bright colors and shapes. They felt that the frequency of such hallucinations was dose related and could be modified by intravenous administration of diazepam.

CARDIOVASCULAR MEDICATIONS

Several agents used for cardiovascular diseases have been reported to produce psychiatric and behavioral disturbances, including hallucinatory symptoms (Paulseth & Klawans, 1985). Digoxin has been implicated by several authors in inducing hallucinations. Closson (1983) noted that visual hallucinations may present as the earliest symptom of digoxin intoxication.

Propranolol, a beta adrenergic blocker, has been associated with lassitude and depression. It has also been described to produce vivid nightmares, hypnagogic hallucinations, and psychosis (Fraser & Carr, 1976). Timolol, another beta adrenergic blocker, was also responsible for inducing syncope and visual hallucinations (Yates, 1980). Clonidine, an alpha adrenergic agonist, was noted to produce hallucinatory symptoms (Brown et al., 1980).

Prazosin, an antihypertensive agent, was noted to induce auditory hallucinations in some patients (Patterson, 1988). Rosenthal (1987) reported a case of an 87-year-old woman who experienced visual hallucinations, depression, and suicidal ideation as a result of taking isosorbide dinitrate, a long-acting vasodilator used for angina. He suggested that the visual hallucinations may be attributed to cerebral ischemia secondary to transient drug-induced hypotension.

Other cardiovascular drugs described to induce visual hallucinations include quinidine, reserpine, methyldopa, and disopyramide (Cummings & Miller, 1987).

ANTINEOPLASTIC AGENTS

Several antineoplastic drugs can cause encephalopathies with resulting psychiatric and behavioral manifestations. Nesse et al. (1983) reported the occurrence of olfactory and gustatory pseudohallucinations in nonpsychotic chemotherapy patients who were in a state of clear consciousness. Patients received a combination of mechlorethamine, vincristine, procarbazine, and prednisone (MOPP). These experiences were closely associated with pretreatment nausea. Walsh et al. (1984) noted that hallucinatory symptoms can occur as an adverse reaction to chlorambucil therapy. Noll and Kulkarni (1984) reported the occurrence of insidious loss of visual acuity and simultaneous onset of complex visual hallucinations in a patient with acute lymphoblastic leukemia, who had recently received bone marrow transplantation and was being treated with prednisone and cyclosporine to suppress graft-v-host disease. Visual hallucinations spontaneously ameliorated with reduction and termination of cyclosporine treatment.

ANTIMICROBIAL AGENTS

Several antibiotics have been associated with psychotic reactions, including hallucinatory symptoms. Robertson (1985) reported the onset of visual hallucinations in a child after receiving a penicillin injection containing 300,000 units of penicillin G procaine and 300,000 units of penicillin G benzathine. Silber and D'Angelo (1985) proposed that hallucinations and seizures associated with procaine penicillin injections may be due to sudden elevation of serum procaine in the central nervous system. Oliver (1984) noted the occurrence of hallucinations in association with amoxycillin treatment. Other antibiotics and antimicrobial agents—including antimalarial agents, cycloserine, isoniazid, sulfonamides, and tetracycline—have been reported to cause visual hallucinations (Cummings & Miller, 1987).

MISCELLANEOUS AGENTS

Cimetidine, the first of a new class of pharmacologic agents that dramatically inhibit the basal gastric acid secretion, has been reported frequently to cause mental confusion and disorientation in patients receiving the drug. Yudofsky et al. (1980) presented three patients who experienced agitation, disorientation, and hallucination while being treated with cimetidine. Papp and Curtis (1984) reported that cimetidine in usual doses can cause visual hallucinations, possibly due to its effect on brain receptors. Ranitidine, a newer H2-receptor antagonist used to inhibit gastric secretion as well, has also been reported to induce mental confusion and hallucinations. Price et al. (1985) presented a case of a 72-year-old female who developed visual hallucinations shortly after initiation of ranitidine therapy. Rechallenge with the drug resulted in both visual and auditory hallucinations following a single dose. The incidence of hallucinatory symptoms that may result from ranitidine therapy appears to be less than that resulting from treatment with cimetidine.

Roy and Wakefield (1986) reported a case of hallucinations following the sudden withdrawal of baclofen, a muscle relaxant and antispastic. Bachman (1984) presented a case of a 77-year-old female who underwent metrizamide myelography of the posterior fossa to elucidate the cause of "downbeat nystagmus." Approximately 12 hours after the procedure, she developed formed visual hallucinations consisting primarily of brightly colored geometric shapes, cloud formations, and human figures. These hallucinations subsided two days later. The author suggested that the visual hallucinations may have been caused by the penetration of the metrizamide into the temporal lobe and visual association cortex.

Other agents reported to induce visual hallucinations include disulfiram (Antabuse), and heavy metals (Cummings & Miller, 1987).

SUMMARY

Several medications and pharmacological agents commonly used in medical practice are capable of inducing various types of psychotic reactions including hallucinations. Visual hallucinations occur more often than other types, and they may or may not be accompanied by delirium. Certain individuals, such as the seriously ill and the elderly, seem to be particularly susceptible to such reactions. These hallucinations generally stop upon the discontinuation of the drug in question. However, the administration of a small dose of a high potency antipsychotic agent may be necessary, especially if the patient needs to be kept on the medication that is causing the hallucinations.

11

Hallucinations Associated with Neurologic Disorders

The correlation between hallucinatory phenomena and central nervous system disease has long been noted by investigators and writers. In fact, some researchers have attempted to induce hallucinatory symptoms by electrical stimulation of various brain structures. Penfield and Rasmussen (1950) succeeded in reproducing visual and auditory hallucinations by electrical stimulation of the temporal lobe cortex. Following that, Mahl et al. (1964) demonstrated that auditory hallucinations can be induced upon stimulation of deep structures of the temporal lobe using a needle electrode. Horowitz and Adams (1970) later produced visual hallucinations by stimulating deep structures of the temporal lobe. They also found that the stimulation of the posterior hippocampus was more likely to result in hallucinatory experiences than the stimulation of any other site.

This type of experimental work suggests that pathological processes leading to anatomical, physiological, and neurochemical changes in specific cerebral areas can lead to hallucinatory experiences. Neurological syndromes that have been described as associated with hallucinations involve epileptic, vascular, neoplastic, traumatic, metabolic, infectious, and other pathological processes.

EPILEPTIC DISORDERS

Persistently or recurrently firing epileptogenic foci may produce hallucinatory phenomena. Hallucinations may be experienced during either the aura or the attack itself. In addition, post-ictal hallucinations have been described. Any sensory modality may be involved depending on the location of the focus. Temporal and occipital lobes are most frequently involved with such epileptic activities. Hallucinatory symptoms may be limited to simple unformed perceptions or they may be more complex and elaborate experiences. In general, it appears that the more posterior the lesion in the temporal cortex, the more complex and structured the hallucinatory experiences (Mayer-Gross et al., 1969)

Complex partial seizures, also known as temporal lobe epilepsy, may be accompanied by schizophrenia-like symptoms in some patients. Psychotic symptoms include a formal thought disorder, delusions, and hallucinations. These psychotic manifestations usually begin several years after the onset of the epilepsy, although some patients become psychotic within a few months of the first seizure (Cummings, 1988). The clinical presentation of complex partial seizures usually involves abrupt onset of "deja vu" or "jamais vu" experiences, perceptual illusions and hallucinations, dream-like sensations, sudden change of emotional tone, aphasia or forced thinking, and automatic repetitive behavior such as lip smacking. The episode terminates abruptly, usually within two minutes, and the patient often recognizes the perceptions as being unreal. Some patients may experience partial loss of consciousness and amnesia (Simonds, 1986). Gillig et al. (1988) reported a case of a patient with right hemisphere complex partial seizures who presented with mania, neologisms, and hallucinations during the ictal periods.

Psychotic symptoms in patients with complex partial seizures are more frequent in females than in males and are more likely to occur in those patients with epileptic foci on the left side of the brain. The psychosis may have an episodic pattern and may decrease as the seizure activity increases in frequency. In fact, controlling the seizure activity in some patients may precipitate a psychotic episode. In such conditions, it was found that psychotic symptoms may improve when anticonvulsant medication is decreased to allow some increase in seizure frequency. Antipsychotic medications seem to have a limited effect in controlling psychotic symptoms associated with complex partial seizures, but occasionally the response may be dramatic (Wells, 1985).

Visual hallucinations occur more frequently than other types of hallucinations in the course of complex partial seizures. Simple unformed visual sensations involving light, darkness, or color are reported most often. However, many patients experience complex dream-like visual hallucinations consisting of complex scenes or pictures. Such perceptions are usually associated with a discharge in the posterior temporal region. Auditory hallucinations are less frequent and may consist of recognizable sounds, music, or voices. These hallucinations are usually associated with a discharge in the superior temporal region.

Olfactory hallucinations often consist of unpleasant odors and occur with a discharge in the uncus, which is located in the anterior mesial part of the temporal lobe; therefore, this type of seizure is often referred to as an uncinate fit. Gustatory hallucinations, consisting of a sensation of abnormal taste, occur with a discharge in the periinsular area (Westmoreland, 1980). Tactile hallucinations are relatively uncommon with temporal lobe epilepsy. Negative hallucinations, in which patients fail to perceive external stimuli, have been described to occur as an ictal phenomenon of partial complex seizures (Keefover et al., 1988).

Hausser and Bancaud (1987) investigated patients with intractable epilepsy and found that four percent manifested gustatory hallucinations as part of their seizures. They noted that gustatory hallucinations occurred in the course of parietal, temporal, or temporoparietal seizures in most of the patients.

Mulder et al. (1957) described a focal type of epilepsy called "hallucinatory epilepsy." In this condition, hallucinations occur abruptly in a paroxysmal fashion. They are usually brief and are followed by a partial impairment of cerebral functioning. During the seizure, there is a stereotypic succession of symptoms in which each component of the hallucination follows another component in a certain order. The same hallucinatory experience tends to be repeated with every episode. Mulder et al. (1957) presented the case of a 43-year-old man who suffered from "hallucinatory epilepsy." The patient described having visual hallucinations that consisted of people who would suddenly appear in front of him, and begin to work and communicate with each other. He added that this experience became a "standardized vision" that occurred during every hallucinatory episode, in the same order and with the same details.

Stacy (1987) described a patient who presented with tactile hallucinations as a clinical manifestation of ictal phenomena.

Occipital lobe epilepsy refers to visual hallucinations in patients with occipital epileptic foci. Strub and Black (1988) noted that posterior lesions of the occipital lobe are associated with simple unformed visual hallucinations such as flashes of light, colors, or spots, whereas more anterior lesions are likely to cause formed and complex visual hallucinations such as images or events. They reported a case of a patient with epileptic foci in the right occipitotemporal region, who developed seizures in the form of hallucinations in the left visual field. The patient experienced himself driving down a road through a forest. Strub and Black (1988) indicated that such "hemihallucinations" are uncommon, but they can be seen in the blind field of some patients with damage to the calcarine cortex. Gastaut and Zifkin (1984) reported three cases of occipital lobe epilepsy in which each patient experienced visual hallucinations of numbers followed by a brief loss of vision during the ictal phase.

Post-ictal phenomena are encountered most commonly in patients with major motor epilepsy. In addition to various physical signs and symptoms, patients exhibit mental confusion, disorientation, and abnormal behavior. In some patients, hallucinations and paranoid ideas may be prominent (Lishman, 1987). Ambrosetto (1986) reported a case of a 32-year-old man with a glioma in the Sylvian region who presented with gustatory hallucinations as a post-ictal symptom.

Another phenomenon that is probably related to seizure activity is known as "palinacousis." This rare condition was described by Jacobs et al. (1973) as recurrent or persistent paroxysmal auditory illusions that may be triggered by environmental stimuli such as voices, music, or other noises. These auditory sensations recur or persist for a variable period of time even after the initial stimulus has subsided, and are usually exact replicas or fragments of the original sound. Malone and Leiman (1983) warned that such hallucinatory experiences could be misdiagnosed as auditory hallucinations of "functional" psychotic illness.

A similar phenomenon, known as "palinopsia," or visual perseveration, also presents with recurrent visual imagery of objects long after they have been removed. Palinopsia is usually associated with CNS pathological processes, such as brain tumors, arteriosclerotic brain disease, and idiopathic epilepsy (Weiner, 1961). This condition should be differentiated from eidetic imagery (see Chapter 13).

BRAIN TUMORS

Brain tumors and other space occupying lesions, such as abscesses and aneurysms, produce certain neurological signs and symptoms depending on their location. Various types of hallucinations have been reported in association with brain tumors. The nature of these hallucinatory symptoms depends on the location of the lesion. Occipital lobe tumors are often associated with unformed visual hallucinations such as flashes of light or colors. Temporal lobe tumors are usually associated with more complex visual hallucinations. In addition, unformed and formed auditory hallucinations as well as gustatory and olfactory hallucinations have been reported in association with temporal lobe tumors. Parietal lobe tumors may produce localized tactile and kinaesthetic hallucinations. Tumors of the frontal lobe sometimes produce visual, auditory, or even gustatory hallucinations, presumably through irritative effects on the neighboring temporal lobe. Furthermore, lesions of the medial aspect of the frontal lobe can discharge directly to the temporal lobe and produce hallucinatory experiences. Subtentorial tumors may compress the adjacent occipital lobe and produce visual hallucinations (Lishman, 1987).

Tumors that compress the optic nerve and optic chiasma have also been reported to cause simple and complex visual hallucinations (Weinberger & Grant, 1940).

Ambrosetto (1986) reported a case of a patient affected by a grade 1 astrocytoma of the right Sylvian region, who presented with epileptic seizures and gustatory hallucinations as a post-ictal symptom. He suggested that post-ictal or ictal gustatory hallucinations may be a localizing symptom of glioma involving the Sylvian region. Dyck (1985) reported a case of a patient who developed auditory hallucinations as a result of a lipoma in the Sylvian region. Vike et al. (1984) described a patient who suffered from a large cystic mass on the left side extending from the medial temporal region to the midbrain. The patient developed a striking auditory-visual synesthesia on the same side of the mass, in which sound stimuli were transformed into visual experiences. Although this type of synesthesia is usually reported in patients with acquired visual loss involving the anterior visual pathways, this patient's neuro-ophthalmologic and neurophysiologic examinations did not disclose any evidence of visual dysfunction. The authors added that the synesthesia disappeared after the mass was excised. Ram et al. (1987) reported three patients with pituitary adenoma whose presenting symptoms were both simple, unformed and complex, formed visual hallucinations. The unformed visual hallucinations were believed to be caused by the compression of the optic nerves and chiasm by the tumor, whereas the complex visual hallucinations were thought to be of the "release" type (see release hallucinations below). Dunn et al. (1983) reported a case of an eight-year-old boy who developed transient visual hallucinations due to extrinsic compression of the midbrain by a cystic craniopharyngioma. The hallucinations resolved promptly after drainage of the cyst.

CEREBROVASCULAR DISEASES

Several investigators have noted the occurrence of psychotic symptoms following strokes. Dunne et al. (1980) reviewed 387 patients who had strokes and found that 19 percent presented exclusively with behavioral alterations and symptoms of delirium, dementia, or delusions.

It had been postulated that there was a specific link between psychosis and right hemispheric dysfunction. However, further studies indicated that both left and right sided temporoparietal strokes may be associated with psychosis (Cummings, 1988).

Hallucinatory symptoms have been described in association with vascular injury or infarction of various areas of the brain. Cogan (1973) described amorphous visual phenomena known as "release" hallucinations caused by damage of the occipital centers. Peroutka et al. (1982) documented the occurrence of formed visual hallucinations and delusions after large temporoparieto-occipital infarction. Tanabe et al. (1986) described a case of a patient who experienced verbal auditory hallucinations lateralized to the right ear and developed fluent aphasia following a hemorrhagic infarction in the left superior temporal gyrus. They concluded that the lateralization phenomenon of complex auditory hallucinations could be considered a significant clinical sign indicating the existence of a lesion in the superior temporal gyrus opposite the hallucination side. Stacy (1987) described a patient with biparietal lesions who demonstrated complex "stereognostic hallucinations" and recurrent tactile sensations. He elaborated that although the patient had suffered from complete astereognosis and palpatory apraxia, he developed hallucinatory experiences in which he described palpating the hallucinated objects appropriately. Pakalnis et al. (1987) reported a case of a patient who developed an agitated psychosis with visual hallucinations and delusional beliefs with a demonstrable lacunar infarction involving the right geniculocalcarine tract. Pardal et al. (1985) reported a case of a hypertensive patient who suffered a right caudate hemorrhage with slight rupture into the ventricular system. The patient experienced hallucinations of an alligator that made unpleasant noises by teeth clenching. The image was vivid and the patient was not aware that it was false. Cascino and Adams (1986) reported the occurrence of auditory hallucinations in three patients with brain stem lesions: two patients had vascular lesions of the tegmentum of the pons and the third had a tumor involving the lower midbrain. Lanska et al. (1987) reported a patient with a caudal pontine hemorrhage who experienced low-pitched, slow musical sounds in both ears. He recognized these sounds as abnormal. Over several days the auditory hallucinations changed into what he described as "like people talking," but he could not make out individual words. Later he heard rain falling on the roof and ringing or clicking noises. The hallucinations resolved over several months. Safran et al. (1981) described a 65-year-old man with ischaemic encephalomalacia following surgery for an aortic arch aneurysm, who experienced episodes of sterotyped formed visual hallucinations uniquely provoked by television viewing.

EXTRAPYRAMIDAL SYNDROMES

Among extrapyramidal syndromes, organic psychosis has been most well documented in Huntington's chorea. A high percentage of patients with Huntington's disease present with psychotic manifestations, mostly delusions, sometimes with Schneiderian first rank symptoms (including auditory hallucinations) and a formal thought disorder (Cummings, 1988).

Parkinson's disease may become complicated with psychotic manifestations at some point during the course of the illness. Lishman (1987) reported that patients with Parkinson's disease may develop changes of personality with suspicion, irritability, egocentricity, and impairment of memory and intellect. In addition, some patients may develop depressive symptoms, paranoid ideation, and sometimes visual hallucinations. Sandyk (1981) noted the occurrence of olfactory hallucinations in the course of Parkinson's disease. In addition, it is important to indicate that several types of hallucinations may occur as a result of treating Parkinson's disease with anticholinergic drugs or dopaminergic agents (Goetz et al., 1982).

Idiopathic basal ganglia calcification (Fahr's disease) was reported to present with Parkinsonian movement disturbance, mild dementia, and, in about 50 percent of patients, with schizophrenia-like psychosis, including persecutory delusions, and auditory and visual hallucinations (Francis, 1979).

Other extrapyramidal syndromes that have been associated with hallucination include Wilson's disease, and Sydenham's chorea or rheumatic chorea (Lishman, 1987).

HEAD INJURIES

Hallucinations have been described in association with head injuries and concussion syndrome (Lishman, 1987). Loyd and Tsuang (1981) reported a case of a patient who developed visual hallucinations of snakes that began ten months after a brief loss of consciousness in a car accident. The patient complained of persistent headaches and depressive symptoms as well. The authors concluded that the hallucinations of snakes might have been a manifestation of post-concussional syndrome. Askenasy et al. (1986) studied patients who suffered missile head injuries during war. Two patients described repetitive visual images during wakefulness when relaxed with closed eyes and also at sleep. The two patients demonstrated diffuse brain lesions, right non-dominant associative area damage, homonymous hemianopia, and post-traumatic stress disorder. The investigators suggested that the presence of PTSD may have contributed to the occurrence of the visual experiences.

MIGRAINE

Migraine headaches are often preceded by visual auras such as scintillating scotomata and may involve unformed visual hallucinations consisting of lines, geometric designs, or mosaics. However, highly complex formed visual hallucinations can occur in certain cases of migraine (Hachinski et al., 1973). In addition, visual distortions including macropsia and micropsia may occur. Wolberg and Ziegler (1982) indicated that migraine headaches may be accompanied by olfactory hallucinations as well.

NARCOLEPSY

Hypnagogic and hypnopompic hallucinations have been reported in cases of narcolepsy. The hallucinations usually have a dream-like quality and involve geometric patterns, landscapes, faces, or figures, and may be associated with visual distortions. Hypnagogic hallucinations are often accompanied by sleep paralysis and are believed to result from the intrusion of dreams of REM sleep into wakefulness (Cummings & Miller, 1987).

Shapiro and Spitz (1976) suggested that patients with narcolepsy who present with hallucinations need to be differentiated from patients with psychotic disorders. In fact, they reported a case of a patient with narcolepsy who presented to the mental hygiene clinic complaining of seeing people in her room and hearing voices "from out of this world." The patient was misdiagnosed as a schizophrenic for some time before the accurate diagnosis of narcolepsy was made.

PEDUNCULAR HALLUCINOSIS

Vascular, neoplastic, or other structural damage of the pons or midbrain may produce a unique type of visual hallucination syndrome known as "peduncular hallucinosis." The condition is usually accompanied by disturbance in the sleep-wake cycle and by cranial nerve palsy. The hallucinations typically occur in the evening and consist of geometric patterns or more complex hallucinations of landscapes, flowers, birds, animals, or people. The patient may react to those experiences with amusement or astonishment and may even look forward to their occurrence (Cummings & Miller, 1987).

RELEASE HALLUCINATIONS

Release hallucinations refer to a certain type of hallucinations that occur when the visual association areas are disconnected from visual input, yet are actively releasing visual images from stored memories (Strub & Black, 1988). Release hallucinations may develop following hemispheric infarctions, tumors, or other destructive lesions of the geniculocalcarine pathways, and they are more common with right-sided than with left-sided lesions. Release hallucinations consist of complex visual images of objects, animals, or people. They can be differentiated from ictal hallucinations by their longer duration (usually hours), their association with visual field defect, and their response to environmental manipulation such as opening, moving, or closing the eyes (Cummings & Miller, 1987).

Lanska et al. (1987) reported a case of a 55-year-old hypertensive man who suffered a left-sided dorsal pontine hemorrhage and small bilateral internal capsule lacunae. Audiometry demonstrated moderate bilateral sensorineural hearing loss with poor speech discrimination on the left. The patient described auditory hallucinations of various sounds that changed over time. The hallucinations eventually resolved over several months. The author suggested that these hallucinations represent release-type phenomena similar to that of the visual release hallucinations.

CENTRAL NERVOUS SYSTEM INFECTIONS

Hallucinations have been reported in the course of various central nervous system infections including herpes encephalitis, Jakob-Creutzfeld disease, tertiary syphilis, and AIDS. Meningitis may present with hallucinatory symptoms as well. These conditions are described in Chapter 8.

METABOLIC AND TOXIC ENCEPHALOPATHIES

Various endocrine disorders such as adrenicortical hypofunction, thyroid disorders, parathyroid disorders, and vitamin D intoxication can result in several psychiatric symptoms including hallucinations. Vitamin deficiency, and electrolyte and mineral disturbances have been known to cause hallucinatory symptoms as well. Hepatic encephalopathy, uremic encephalopathy, and porphyria can produce hallucinations. In addition, intoxication with various chemical agents and poisons such as carbon dioxide, mercury, and bromide can lead to delirious states with hallucinations. These conditions are discussed in Chapter 8.

DEMENTIAS

Various types of hallucinatory symptoms have been described in patients with Alzheimer's disease and multi-infarct dementia. Details of such phenomena are provided in Chapter 8.

HALLUCINATIONS IN OTHER NEUROLOGICAL CONDITIONS

Aqueduct stenosis has been reported to manifest with psychotic symptoms. Roberts et al. (1983) presented the case histories of five adult patients with hydrocephalus and aqueduct stenosis. All cases were associated with prominent delusions, hallucinations, or thought disorder. All five patients were classified as schizophrenics. The authors suggested that dysfunction in subcortical structures, notably the mesencephalic regions of the brain, could have played an important role in the etiology of the schizophrenic psychoses in such individuals. They added that it is possible that intrinsic brain-stem pathology might be responsible for aqueduct stenosis and also for the associated psychosis.

Auditory hallucinations have been reported in some patients with atypical tic disorder. Kerbeshian and Burd (1985) presented two patients with such conditions. The first patient was a 10-year-old boy who had attention deficit disorder with hyperactivity and atypical tic disorder. He reported command auditory hallucinations giving him mundane orders such as "carry out the trash" or "clean your room." The second patient was a 15-year-old boy with atypical tic disorder with probable attention deficit disorder without hyperactivity. He experienced auditory hallucinations during the day and at night when he was ready to go to bed, but well in advance of his going to sleep. The voices usually evaluated the patient's recent activities in a negative light. The authors hypothesized that these auditory experiences represented increased and intense auditory receptiveness which might reflect auditory perceptual hypersensitivity.

Other neurological conditions that have been reported to be associated with hallucinatory symptoms include: multiple sclerosis, diffuse cerebral sclerosis, Friedreich's ataxia, normal pressure hydrocephalus, temporal arteritis, periarteritis nodosa involving cerebral blood vessels, and systemic lupus erythematosis with CNS involvement (Lishman, 1987).

SUMMARY

Various types of simple or complex hallucinations can occur in association with different neurological disorders. The nature of the hallucinatory experience is largely dependent on the anatomical location of the lesion and the underlying organic pathology. In general, such hallucinations are recognized by the individual as unreal. The treatment should be directed at the underlying disorder, however, symptomatic treatment may be required.

12 =

Hallucinations Associated With Ear and Eye Diseases

Auditory hallucinations have been reported in patients with partial or complete hearing loss. Similarly, visual hallucinations occur in patients with partial or complete blindness. It is generally believed that hallucinatory phenomena experienced in such conditions are largely due to sensory deprivation. Hallucinations reported under these circumstances can vary from simple unformed perceptions to highly complex formed hallucinatory experiences. Individuals usually recognize these perceptions as being unreal, and therefore, they may be referred to as pseudohallucinations.

EAR DISEASES

Auditory hallucinations are known to occur in individuals with acquired hearing loss. However, there is some evidence in the literature that prelingually deaf people are capable of experiencing auditory hallucinations. In addition, it has been noted that schizophrenic patients who suffer from variable degrees of hearing loss, including complete deafness, have reported several forms of auditory hallucinations.

Hallucinations in People with Acquired Deafness

Hammeke et al. (1983) described two patients with a long history of progressive bilateral hearing loss, who experienced auditory hallucinations that varied from simple unformed auditory perceptions, such as tinnitus and irregular sounds, to complex formed auditory hallucinations of instrumental music, singing, and voices. The authors emphasized that the patients did not show any evidence of global dementia, epileptic disturbance, or psychiatric disorders that might account for the hallucinatory symptoms. Rosanski and Rosen (1952) indicated that patients with progressive hearing loss due to otosclerosis have reported experiencing musical hallucinations. Raghuram et al. (1980) noted the occurrence of similar musical hallucinations in a 52-year-old man who had suffered progressive bilateral sensori-neural hearing loss over 40 years.

As indicated earlier, it is believed that prolonged sensory deprivation plays an essential role in the etiology of hallucinatory phenomena associated with acquired deafness, however, a recent report by Aizenberg et al. (1986) argued that depression might have a contributory role in such instances as well. The authors noted that musical hallucinations associated with acquired deafness were rarely reported in the psychiatric literature, and, in the few cases studied, no evidence of psychiatric disturbance was found. They described two patients who experienced musical hallucinations during a state of nonpsychotic depression. One of the two patients suffered from acquired deafness. The other patient did not demonstrate any organic pathology. The authors concluded that musical hallucinations stopped concomitantly in both patients with the improvement of their affective state.

In any event, it is important to keep in mind that auditory hallucinations in individuals with acquired deafness may be caused by primary psychiatric disorders or other organic conditions. Such disorders need to be ruled out before the final diagnosis is made. Furthermore, and as indicated earlier by Aizenberg et al. (1986), the presence of other psychiatric or organic conditions in such individuals is likely to exacerbate the hallucinatory syndrome.

Hallucinations in Prelingually Deaf Individuals

The question of whether auditory hallucinations require an intact hearing sense at birth, or they may occur in prelingually deaf people has intrigued many researchers and observers for many years. Until the present date, this issue remains controversial despite the fact that, over the past hundred years, several cases of auditory hallucinations have been reported to occur in prelingually deaf individuals.

The earliest case was noted by Stearns (1886) who described a "deaf mute" woman with "folie circulaire" who experienced auditory hallucinations. More recently, Rainer et al. (1970) conducted an extensive research with deaf psychiatric patients and demonstrated that auditory hallucinations could, in fact, occur in prelingually deaf patients, in addition to visual hallucinations. They reported several cases to illustrate that point. One patient, who had become deaf at the age of one year, and who was married to a deaf woman, developed schizophrenia and said that he heard the voice of God. The patient drew a picture of himself surrounded by words entering his body via wires through his ears. The authors reported several other patients who were born deaf and experienced auditory hallucinations of various kinds during the course of their psychiatric illnesses.

Altshuler (1971) reported observations extending over 16 years of schizophrenic patients with early total deafness. He noted that auditory hallucinations occurred in about the same proportion of those individuals as in schizophrenics with intact hearing sense. He found that 22 of 57 deaf schizophrenics had hallucinations. Seventeen of these patients described "some sort of auditory phenomena." He suggested that these observations support the theory that auditory hallucinations are produced by a "central organic mechanism."

Evans and Elliot (1981) studied 13 psychotic deaf patients for the diagnosis of schizophrenia. Most patients reported hallucinatory experiences consisting mainly of visual, tactile, and somatic types. Auditory hallucinations were reported only in those patients who, at some point in their lives, had experienced sound to some degree.

Critchley et al. (1981) studied 12 prelingually profoundly deaf schizophrenic adults. The authors reported that visual hallucinations occurred in 10 patients. They also noted that these patients had experiences "analogous to auditory hallucinations, although voices may not have been heard." The authors concluded that these observations may be taken as supportive of the concept of a "nuclear form" of schizophrenia and raise interesting points concerning the relationship between thought process and language.

A recent report by Harry and Favazza (1984) described a 31-year-old prelingually deaf man who developed a brief reactive psychosis during which he experienced auditory and visual hallucinations of the devil and God "pulling" and threatening him. He reported to the staff, using American Sign Language, that the devil told him to commit suicide. The psychotic symptoms resolved rapidly after proper intervention. The author suggested that the auditory hallucinations fulfilled his wishes to gain his hearing, and the visual hallucinations "symbolically anchored him to the predominantly visual world of the nonhearing."

EYE DISEASES

Visual hallucinations have been reported in several ophthalmologic disorders affecting the visual apparatus and leading to partial or complete blindness. These disorders include: injury to the globe, cataract formation, glaucoma, macular degeneration, retinal disease, and optic nerve disease. It is believed that prolonged visual sensory deprivation plays a significant role in the emergence of visual hallucinations in patients with blindness. Visual hallucinatory symptoms associated with eye disease may be complex or simple, depending on the underlying ophthalmologic disease. Hallucinations that occur after progressive cataract formation that leads to blindness tend to be formed and complex, whereas those hallucinations resulting from retinal diseases, optic nerve diseases, and glaucoma are mostly simple and unformed. Most patients when experiencing these hallucinations are fully aware of the unreality of their perceptions (Cummings & Miller, 1987).

Visual Hallucinations in Cataract

Complex formed visual hallucinations are known to occur in association with cataracts (Bartlett, 1951). Levine (1980) reported the cases of two elderly patients with dense, bilateral cataracts who experienced vivid and intense complex visual hallucinations consisting of people, brightly colored flowers, and other objects. The experiences were usually of a short duration, lasting seconds or a few minutes at most, and occurred daily for months. The majority of the hallucinations were pleasant and beautiful, and the patients were able to describe them to the smallest detail. The patients were fully alert, oriented, and aware that the hallucinations were unreal. These visual hallucinations disappeared following surgical cataract extraction.

Levine (1980) also noted that visual hallucinations may develop postoperatively following cataract extraction in certain patients who did not have such experiences before the surgery. He suggested that the postoperative hallucinations in such cases may include both visual and auditory types, as well as paranoid delusions and behavioral disturbances. Such hallucinations are clearly different from preoperative hallucinations and may represent delirious postoperative complications.

Olbrich et al. (1987) studied 43 patients with severe visual impairment due to bilateral eye disease. Twenty-eight patients underwent eye surgery. Three of the 28 patients had no previous history of halucinatory phenomena, however, they experienced visual hallucinations on the second day after surgery without showing any other psychiatric symptoms.

Visual Hallucinations Associated with Retinal Diseases and Glaucoma

Brief simple visual hallucinations consisting of flashes of light may be induced by retinal traction secondary to retinal detachment. Simple visual hallucinations of rainbows surrounding objects have been described by patients with acute glaucoma due to a sudden increase in intraocular pressure (Cummings & Miller, 1987).

Complex visual hallucinations may occur in patients with partial blindness due to retinal disease. White (1980) reported two patients who had macular degeneration, and a third who had choroideraemia. The patients experienced complex, formed, visual hallucinations consisting of brightly colored stereotyped figures, animals, and objects. The hallucinations began abruptly and appeared to be provoked by light. The patients noted that as the blindness progressed, the clarity, frequency, and duration of the hallucinations faded.

A recent report by Adair and Keshavan (1988) described an elderly patient who had become blind secondary to bilateral glaucoma eight years previously. The patient developed visual hallucinations one month following the death of her son. She began to experience nightly visions of him and other deceased relatives whom she would see in detail. The authors suggested that though sensory deprivation had contributed to the hallucinatory experience, grief reaction might have caused a compensatory recall of visual memory traces and manifested with visual hallucinations. This suggestion was supported by the observation that after proper grief work in which the patient was encouraged to talk about her losses and about her grief for her son, her hallucinations ceased within several weeks.

Visual Hallucinations Associated with Optic Neuritis

Optic nerve disease may give rise to unformed visual hallucinations when the nerve is inflamed. Davis et al. (1976) reported the occurrence of fleeting, bright flashes of light (known as "phosphenes") in patients with optic neuritis and multiple sclerosis. The hallucinations were induced almost exclusively by eye movement and were best perceived in a dark room or in a dimly lit room with the eyes closed. The flashes of light were very brief and lasted for one or two seconds. The phenomenon could be temporarily fatigued by repeated eye movements, but it reappeared after several minutes of rest. The authors emphasized that these phosphenes were distinguished from other phosphenes elicited by eye movements or by pressing or rubbing the optic globe in normal individuals, and from those seen in cases associated with vitreous opacities, in which vitreous "floaters" are nearly always seen. These floaters are believed to result from degenerative changes and vitreous retraction with subsequent tugging on the peripheral retina (Davis et al. 1976).

Patients with visual loss due to lesions of the optic nerve or chiasm were reported to experience unformed and semiformed visual hallucinations when startled by sound. Jacobs et al. (1981) described nine such patients who suffered from optic neuritis, optic chiasm tumors, and optic nerve vascular disorders. Descriptions of the visual experiences varied from simple flashes of white light to complicated colorful hallucinations of various shapes, which always appeared within a defective portion of the visual field. These hallucinations were provoked by sounds of normal daily life that ranged from soft to loud. The sounds always seemed to be heard by the ear ipsilateral to the eye in which the visual experience was produced. The authors concluded that this auditory-visual synesthesia had resulted from postdenervation supersensitivity of the lateral geniculate neurons. Vike et al. (1984) reported a similar patient who developed a striking auditory-visual synesthesia ipsilateral to a large mass involving the medial temporal lobe and the adjacent midbrain. The patient did not show any evidence of visual dysfunction based on neurophthalmologic and neurophysiologic examinations. The authors noted that the synesthesia disappeared after the removal of the mass. They concluded that auditory-visual synesthesia occurred because of direct irritation or deafferentation of "bimodal" neurons that serve to transmit both auditory and visual stimuli within the brain stem.

Charles Bonnet Syndrome

Originally described by Charles Bonnet in 1769, this syndrome refers to the occurrence of vivid, elaborate and well organized visual hallucinations in the elderly. The patients are usually conscious with intact intellectual competence and are fully aware of the unreality of the experiences. Peripheral ocular pathology may be present or absent. The hallucinations involve changing scenes of trees, flowers, buildings, or persons. The experiences usually persist for seconds or hours at a time, and the patient sometimes greets such phenomena with surprise, curiosity, or delight. The hallucinations may disappear or persist when the eyes are closed. The syndrome was formerly thought to be of an idiopathic origin, however, it is currently believed that occult ocular pathologic disorders contribute to most cases (Damas-Mora et al., 1982; Berrios & Brook, 1982).

McNamara et al. (1982) reported a 64-year-old woman who developed complex visual hallucinations that consisted of snakes crawling out of people's heads and onto her body. The patient had become blind 14 years prior to the onset of the hallucinations due to a large suprasellar meningioma. Surgical removal of the tumor was followed by disappearance of the hallucination. The authors suggested that these hallucinations were of the "release" type (see Chapter 11), and were related to both sensory deprivation and impairment in CNS functioning.

Rosenbaum et al. (1987) described two patients with Charles Bonnet syndrome who experienced well organized, clearly defined, vivid visual hallucinations of people and objects. One patient had dense bilateral cataracts, and the other suffered from pigmentary macular degeneration in both eyes. The authors warned that elderly patients who present with visual hallucinations may be misdiagnosed and dismissed as being demented or psychotic because this syndrome is not well recognized in clinical practice. They presented several theories to explain this phenomenon. The sensory deprivation theory holds that removal of normal visual impulses leads to the "release" of indigenous cerebral activity of the visual system in the form of hallucinations. The irritative focus model suggests that the cells of the visual association cortex are more likely to discharge spontaneously when normal afferent input is reduced. This concept is supported by the fact that complex visual hallucinations in the course of Charles Bonnet syndrome occur episodically rather than continuously, and that anticonvulsant medications may reduce or abolish these hallucinations.

A third view suggests a psychologic etiology in which the visual hallucinations are believed to represent a highly complex psychological synthesis resulting from integrative activities of the mind that fuse memory, factual associations, and previous visual experiences with simple sensory presentations to create an image.

Anton's Syndrome

Anton's syndrome refers to a condition in which the patient who suffers from acquired blindness denies blindness and attempts to behave as though he or she can see, and then describes purely imaginary visual experiences when tested. The syndrome is especially present when blindness is due to lesions of the optic radiations or striate cortices (Lishman, 1987). The visual hallucinations and the denial of blindness appear to be transient and usually decrease over time (Strub & Black, 1988).

Entoptic Phenomena

The entoptic phenomena refer to the visualization of certain structures within the eye through the proper arrangement of incident light. These structures may include floaters, which consist of translucent specks of various shapes and sizes that float across the visual field. These structures may be normal, or they may be imperfections such as opacities in the vitreous or the lens. The structures can be seen only when the eye is open (Moses, 1981). "Scheerer's phenomenon" is an entoptic phenomenon in which the person visualizes red blood cells circulating in the paramacular region of the retina. This phenomenon occurs in association with circulation disturbances of the retina (Priestley & Foree, 1955).

Phantom Vision

Hallucinations associated with blindness are sometimes known as "phantom vision" to emphasize their similarity to "phantom limb syndrome." Phantom visions may occur in patients who have suffered traumatic enucleation of one or both eyes, and appear to be behaviorally related to the somatosensory phenomenon of "phantom limb syndrome" in which the person may still feel the extremity after it has been amputated (Cohn, 1971).

SUMMARY

Simple and complex auditory hallucinations have been reported by individuals suffering from complete or partial hearing loss. Such experiences are largely due to prolonged sensory deprivation. In addition, there is some evidence that auditory hallucinations can occur in prelingually deaf individuals.

Similarly, simple and complex visual hallucinations can follow partial or complete blindness resulting from various ophthalmological disorders. Sensory deprivation and other mechanisms have been implicated in such conditions.

13 ═══

Hallucinations in Children

Hallucinatory symptoms are relatively uncommon among child psychiatric patients. As reported by various studies, the frequency of occurrence of hallucinations in that population ranges from 0.4 percent to 5.7 percent. Hallucinations in children are mostly of the auditory modality, however, other types occur as well. It has been suggested that some hallucinatory experiences in children may represent a normal maturational phenomenon, in the absence of any organic pathology or psychosis. Such "nonmorbid" hallucinations should be differentiated from other types that occur in the course of psychiatric or organic conditions such as schizophrenia, depression, anxiety, phobia, drug toxicity, metabolic disorders, infections, or seizure disorders (Kotsopoulos et al., 1987).

DEVELOPMENTAL CONSIDERATIONS

The mental life of children is rich with fantasies and imagination. In fact, the distinction between fantasy and reality in the child's mind may be blurred. There is some disagreement among writers as to the age at which the child is able to make such a distinction. However, it has been suggested that children's preoccupation with fantasies and imaginary activities may actually foster their adaptation to reality (Pilowsky & Chambers, 1986).

According to Piaget (1962), until the age of three years old, the child still cannot distinguish between dreams and reality. After that age, he or she becomes able to realize that dreams are not real, but believes that they exist in the room as visible pictures. This continues until about age six, after which the child discovers that dreams do not exist in the external world, and that they are products of one's mind. Pilowsky (1986a) made a parallel between the dream/reality distinction and the hallucination/fantasy distinction and questioned, based on Piaget's work, whether the term "hallucination" can be applied in a meaningful way before the age of six.

Piaget (1962) added that the child between four and six years of age is mostly "egocentric" and fails to take into account the point of view of people around him or her. The child at this age may talk about products of his or her imagination, but may not refer to their imaginary nature, even though he or she is aware of that fact.

Pilowsky and Chambers (1986) emphasized that it is important to avoid labeling a child's experience as hallucinatory when the child is experiencing normal developmental phenomena. On the other hand, they noted that the clinician may be led to believe that a child is experiencing normal developmental phenomena when, in fact, the child is actually hallucinating.

HALLUCINATIONS AND THE MATURATION PROCESS IN CHILDREN

Bender (1970) suggested that hallucinations in children have a maturational pattern and may be affected by disturbances or lags in the maturation processes. She argued that children three to six years of age have hallucinatory experiences that are different from those of older children. These hallucinations consist mostly of seeing or hearing imaginary companions. Bender (1970) viewed this phenomenon as a normal dynamic process in the development of the personality, though it seems to occur more commonly among deprived, lonely, or highly imaginative and gifted children, and in children who have special problems in identity or interpersonal relationships. Such experiences may continue into later childhood to fulfill a need and compensate for deficiency in emotional and social experiences.

Bender (1970) noted that children three to six years of age may also experience hallucinatory symptoms in certain organic states such as intoxications with medications and severe infections, or in response to severe emotional stress. Under such pathological conditions, hallucinations may be experienced as frightening animals such as snakes, rats, alligators, or other animals that may be seen as ready to attack the child.

According to Bender (1970), the hallucinations of children from six to 12 years of age have certain characteristics that differentiate them from those of adults. They mostly represent introjected objects or voices of good and bad entities, and are rarely projected to the outside world as in adults. The voices heard by the child serve to direct his or her impulses and are recognized by the child as being unreal and as originating from his or her own individual experiences. These hallucinations usually disappear or fade away as the child approaches puberty or early adolescence.

Bender (1970) added that adolescent hallucinations usually resemble those of adults, but some adolescents may continue to have childish hallucinatory experiences throughout adolescence. She emphasized that childhood hallucinations that occur as part of maturational experiences should be distinguished from hallucinations experienced by schizophrenic children which are usually "of bizarre and richly fanciful nature."

In all events, hallucinatory experiences in children, at whatever age they may occur, should always be viewed as a useful tool to explore the inner world of the child in order to understand his or her complex unconscious psychodynamic issues.

Eidetic Imagery

Weiner (1961) defined eidetic imagery as "the recurrence of a sensation or perception after removal of the perceived object, whether the object be perceived visually or by any other modality." He added that an eidetic individual is capable of reexperiencing the visual imagery of an object shortly after it is removed, but recurrence of vivid imagery may still be experienced after as long as several years.

Eidetic imagery may be present at any age, however, the incidence seems to decrease as one grows older. This condition is fairly common in preschool children with no demonstrable neurotic symptoms or emotional maladjustment. The child is usually aware of the unreality of the experiences (Pilowsky, 1986a). The eidetic imagery phenomenon normally disappears by puberty.

A similar phenomenon, known as "palinopsia," or visual perseveration, also presents with recurrent visual imagery and should be differentiated from eidetic imagery. Palinopsia occurs in adults and is usually associated with CNS pathological processes such as brain tumors, arteriosclerotic brain disease, and idiopathic epilepsy (Weiner, 1961).

Imaginary Companions

Some children describe clear images of people or objects as imaginary companions with whom they play and whom they treat as real, but the child recognizes that the object does not exist in reality (Egdell & Kolven, 1972). This phenomenon is most common in children between three and five years of age. The child plays with the hallucinated companion and may provide sleeping space and a place at the table for the imaginary friend (Bender, 1954).

Imaginary companions are often found in nonpsychotic children, with the highest incidence being among lonely individuals. Some investigators have reported that this phenomenon is particularly common in children who are more intelligent or more creative than others, however, these views remain controversial. In all events, the phenomenon is considered normal by most authors (Pilowsky, 1986a).

It is clear that these imaginary play objects and companions serve to fulfill a need in the child's life and may compensate for deficiency in his or her social and environmental experiences (Bender, 1970). Taken within this context, imaginary companions may be viewed as transitional objects that can help the child develop the capacity for object constancy.

Although this phenomenon is usually found in children from three to five years of age, and is expected to fade away as the child reaches puberty, there are some reports indicating that imaginary companions have been described by nonpsychotic individuals who were college students (Weiner, 1961).

HALLUCINATIONS IN PHOBIC AND ANXIETY DISORDERS

Children who are subjected to severe stress that may be associated with overwhelming anxiety or acute phobic reactions may experience hallucinatory symptoms. A child who is afraid of the dark may experience severe anxiety when subjected to such situations and may report seeing staring eyes or glaring mythical animals (Simonds, 1986).

Kostopoulos et al. (1987) studied 11 nonpsychotic children who experienced hallucinations and found that three of them had primary anxiety disorder and five others had adjustment disorder with anxiety. The ages of the patients ranged from seven to 12 years. The children reported complex auditory hallucinations consisting of various voices telling them mostly frightening things, and formed visual hallucinations consisting of scary scenes. The hallucinations occurred mostly at bedtime, however, the authors did not consider these experiences to be related to hypnagogic or hypnopompic phenomena. Most children were substantially impaired as indicated by the scale of adaptive functioning, and they were either socially inept or withdrawn. The authors added that these hallucinations ceased early in the course of the treatment in most of the cases.

Schreier and Libow (1986) described the occurrence of acute phobic hallucinations in children between two and six years of age. They reported six cases in which children experienced hallucinatory symptoms in response to extreme stressful situations resulting in severe anxiety and phobic behavior. The hallucinations were mostly visual or tactile. They were self limited and lasted for a few days. All children returned to normal functioning after appropriate therapeutic interventions were taken.

Children who experience post-traumatic stress disorder may report hallucinatory symptoms. Simonds (1986) noted that some children who witnessed horrifying events such as rape, homicide, or suicide may have hallucinations in the form of recurrent intense perceptual experiences and intrusive images related to the traumatic events.

HALLUCINATIONS IN DEPRESSED CHILDREN

Chambers (1986) noted that affective disorders in children may present with significant psychotic features including hallucinations and delusions. In fact, he reviewed several studies that investigated childhood psychosis and concluded that some of the children who had been diagnosed as schizophrenics may have had psychotic forms of affective disorders.

Kotsopoulos et al. (1987) reported several cases of hallucinatory symptoms in children with various psychiatric diagnoses. Two children were diagnosed as having adjustment disorder with depressed mood. An eight-year-old girl reported depressive symptoms including sleep disturbance and suicidal ideation. She experienced auditory hallucinations of voices urging her to "go to the knives" and kill herself. The voices were heard while the child was in bed, in the evening or morning, and could "awaken" her from her sleep and "continue to talk." The second child, a 12-year-old boy with depressive symptoms, also reported auditory hallucinations of voices of bad people or the devil urging him to be aggressive and to "retaliate." The voices occurred in school and at home. The child experienced nightmares, sleep talking, and screaming episodes as well.

Simonds (1986) described a case of auditory hallucinations related to depression and grief. He reported a 12-year-old girl who became depressed and anxious after starting junior high school. Her depression was related to several stressors and to unresolved grief over the sudden death of her stepfather. The child began experiencing a human voice telling her to kill herself by overdosing on aspirin.

HALLUCINATIONS IN SCHIZOPHRENIC CHILDREN

Children who fulfill the diagnostic criteria for schizophrenia may present with hallucinatory symptoms similar to those reported by adult schizophrenics. All sensory modalities may be involved, although auditory and visual types are more common. Portell (1970) described hallucinations in preadolescent schizophrenic children. He noted that the frequency of the auditory hallucinations was more than double that of the visual ones. Some children reported hearing frightening voices of a distant figure such as God, a dead person, or a domineering parent commanding fear and anxiety. The visual hallucinations were less vivid, but involved seeing frightening images of the devil, a man without a head, or monsters. Those children were socially isolated and withdrawn.

Hallucinations arising in the course of schizophrenic disorders in children may be differentiated from hallucinations of other psychiatric or organic disorders by their bizarre nature and the presence of other schizophrenic symptoms.

HALLUCINATIONS IN CHILDREN WITH ORGANIC
MENTAL DISORDERS

Organic mental disorders in children occasionally present with hallucinatory symptoms. Severe infection with elevated temperature may lead to delirious states with clouding of consciousness, disorientation, restlessness, severe anxiety, and hallucinations, especially of the visual type. Most childhood infectious diseases have been reported to produce delirious states that can last for several hours to a week. Hallucinatory symptoms associated with delirious states have been reported in cases of CNS infections such as meningitis, encephalitis, brain abscess, rheumatic fever encephalitis, porphyria, uremia, and diabetes mellitus. Furthermore, delirium in children may result from nutritional deficiencies associated with starvation and chronic debilitating diseases.

In addition, delirium in children may be caused by toxic reactions to drugs or other chemicals. Some of the medications commonly given to children that are implicated in the production of hallucinatory symptoms include Ritalin and amphetamine (Paulseth & Klawans, 1985), atropine and similar anticholinergic preparations (Weiner, 1961), antihistamines and decongestants that are present in most cough and cold medicines (Woodward & Baldassano, 1988; Sankey et al., 1984; Dungal, 1984), penicillin (Robertson, 1985) and amoxycillin (Oliver, 1984). Other medications that have been reported to produce hallucinations include barbiturates, Dilantin, and aspirin (Weiner, 1961).

Organic mental disorders in children that also may present with hallucinatory symptoms include migraine, epilepsy, narcolepsy, brain tumors, and other intracranial pathological conditions. Hallucinations associated with organic mental disorders are discussed in detail in Chapter 8.

HALLUCINATIONS IN OTHER CONDITIONS

Hallucinations may be present in association with certain cultural and environmental circumstances. Examples include parents with superstitious beliefs or mystical religions. In such instances the child may use hallucinations in order to elicit attention from the parents (Simonds, 1986). Bender and Lipkowitz (1940) described the case of a nine-year-old boy who reported auditory and visual hallucinations consisting of hearing voices like spirits calling him and seeing lions on the street. These hallucinations were encouraged by his parents who thought that the child had a special gift. The child carried out his hallucinatory experiences as a way to obtain further attention from his parents.

It has been suggested that hallucinations are more frequent in deprived, low-income families (Wilking & Paoli, 1966). Rothstein (1981) argued that several factors may contribute to the production of hallucinatory phenomena in children in this population including emotional deprivation, overstimulation, and neglect.

Hallucinatory experiences have been described in children in the course of dissociative disorders, following sleep deprivation and sensory deprivation (Simonds, 1986).

DIAGNOSTIC CONSIDERATIONS

One of the major difficulties in assessing hallucinatory symptoms in children is determining whether the child is actually hallucinating or is simply experiencing vivid imagery and fantasies. This becomes particularly difficult when the child is under six years of age. In addition, once it is established that the child is hallucinating, it becomes essential to determine how to view such psychotic manifestations with regard to treatment implications and prognosis. Apart from the fact that young children may not be able to provide accurate symptom descriptions essential for accurate diagnosis, some hallucinatory symptoms are viewed as normal developmental phenomena as noted earlier. It is important to emphasize that the presence of hallucinations in adults does not necessarily imply psychotic conditions, but this is even more true in children as they are more likely to present with hallucinatory symptoms in the absence of psychotic disorders.

Pilowsky (1986a) suggested that in order to assess the presence of hallucinations in children, it is important to have the clinician observe the child to evaluate the child's degree of involvement with internal stimuli and the degree of interference with reality testing, adaptation, and judgment; i.e., whether the child believes that the hallucinations represent real objects and whether he or she acts on them. In addition, it is essential to obtain detailed psychiatric history from the child and, especially, from the family. Pilowsky (1986a) stressed that the clinician must avoid putting words into the child's mouth, but at the same time, make sure that the child understands the differences among dreams, daydreams, imagery, and hallucinations. The way the question is presented to the child and the sequence of the proper questions are extremely important in clinical assessment of hallucinations in children. Additionally, the clinician must look for other psychiatric symptoms such as bizarre delusions and should assess the child's affect with regard to its range and appropriateness. The presence of acute anxiety, phobia, or depression should be taken into account in making a clinical assessment as well. Furthermore, it is necessary to conduct a thorough physical examination and appropriate medical work-up to rule out any organic condition that might be responsible for the hallucinatory symptoms.

Rothstein (1981) presented several clinical guidelines that may aid the clinician in making the proper diagnosis and in assessing the prognostic significance of hallucinatory symptoms in children. He noted that, generally, older children who hallucinate may have a worse prognosis than those of younger age. Lags in developmental and intellectual functions may worsen the child's reality testing. The child who cannot recognize the unreality of the hallucinatory experiences readily and who may be quite involved in them, may have a poorer prognosis. Finally, the child's general level of functioning and of emotional and social adaptation are of major significance in determining the long-term prognosis.

Of relevance to the diagnostic issue is a recent study by Burke et al. (1985) that assessed psychopathology in relatives of children with hallucinations. The authors noted that both psychotic and nonpsychotic children who reported hallucinations had significantly more relatives with a history of psychosis as compared to the controls. The psychoses were most likely schizophrenia, schizoaffective disorders, and manic depressive disorders. Furthermore, hallucinating children frequently showed a positive family history of depression; particularly, a depressed mother. However, they did not differ from the control group in this respect.

PSYCHODYNAMIC SIGNIFICANCE OF HALLUCINATIONS IN CHILDREN

Regardless of the etiology of hallucinatory experiences, it is extremely important to understand the underlying psychodynamic factors involved in the condition. These psychodynamic factors provide a very useful tool in order to uncover unconscious conflicts and to work with the child towards recovery.

Hallucinations may be viewed at times as a way to modify harsh realities or as an escape mechanism. Often hallucinatory experiences serve to satisfy wishes and fantasies, such as the desire for enhancing self-esteem or experiencing pleasure. In addition, hallucinations may be regarded as a way of projecting anxiety to an external concrete source where it can be experienced as coming from the outside, instead of feeling it internally. Hostility can be defended against by projecting angry impulses and then reexperiencing them in the form of angry voices coming from the outside. Some hallucinations help to alleviate guilt or shame. Sometimes hallucinations provide an opportunity to reexperience past happy events, or even past traumatic events in order to give the child further opportunity to work out unconscious emotional conflicts (Simonds, 1986).

Pilowsky (1986b) reviewed psychoanalytic theories as they apply to hallucinatory phenomena. He noted that hallucinations may be considered as an expression of superego function. In this context, hearing critical or censuring voices indicates the presence of a punitive, rigid, and primitive superego. When the parents are very critical and abusive, hallucinations may represent the internalization of punitive parental object. Pilowsky (1986b) added that hallucinations may also be viewed as an expression of ego function or id function. As an expression of ego function, the voices reflect attempts to achieve mastery or gain satisfaction in adaptive or partially adaptive ways. As an expression of id function, hallucinations may represent the projection of unacceptable sexual and aggressive impulses. Finally, Pilowsky (1986b) argued that from the object relation viewpoint, hallucinatory experiences may be seen as an expression of internalized objects; and from the interpersonal perspective, hallucinations may be seen as representations of past or current interpersonal experiences. Psychodynamic theories of hallucinations are discussed in Chapter 5.

SUMMARY

Hallucinations in children can be viewed as normal developmental phenomena that serve to fulfill certain needs or compensate for deficiency in emotional and social experiences. However, true hallucinations can occur in children who are suffering from anxiety, depression, or schizophrenic disorders. Furthermore, hallucinations in children can be induced by a wide variety of organic conditions. Differential diagnosis is essential in order to provide appropriate treatment and assess prognostic implications.

14

Hypnosis, Suggestions, and Dissociative States

Various types of hallucinatory symptoms may be induced in some people who are under the influence of a strong suggestion or hypnosis. They can also occur in certain individuals during dissociative states. It is believed that altered states of consciousness weaken the integrative function of the ego and impair the sense of reality, allowing the unconscious material to be projected, and hence become readily available to the person's sensory perception. In this context, hallucinatory phenomena that occur during altered states of consciousness are viewed as a mechanism that serves to facilitate the expression of unconscious conflicts or the fulfillment of certain needs.

HALLUCINATIONS INDUCED BY HYPNOSIS AND SUGGESTIONS

Alexander (1970) defined hypnosis as "a state manifested by an inward turning of the mind, facilitating the enhancement of the creative imagination." He added that under hypnosis, and with appropriate suggestions, the need for reality testing is reduced, providing a mental setting in which ideas can be perceived and experienced in such a vivid manner to the point of actual hallucinations. Alexander (1970) pointed out that hallucinatory experiences induced under hypnosis can be utilized to uncover important unconscious psychodynamic issues and to facilitate therapeutic interventions. He argued that specific "therapeutic hallucinations" may be induced in order to help patients overcome certain psychological conflicts, such as phobic reactions, by working through the anxieties that arise during the "hallucinatory re-vivification of the feared stressful situation."

Barber (1970) reviewed three experiments done on students who reported experiencing auditory and visual hallucinations under hypnotic suggestion. In those experiments half of the subjects clearly heard the suggested sounds, and nearly one-third of them clearly saw the suggested objects.

Young et al. (1987) investigated the role of brief instructions and suggestibility in the elicitation of auditory and visual hallucinations in normal and psychiatric subjects. They compared a group of normal subjects who were predisposed to hallucinate with another group of normal individuals who were not predisposed to such phenomena, as assessed by the Launay-Slade Hallucination Scale (LSHS-A). They also compared a group of hallucinating psychiatric patients with another group of psychiatric patients with no hallucinatory symptoms. The authors found that both the normal individuals who were predisposed to hallucinate, as well as hallucinating psychiatric patients, were significantly more likely to hear suggested sounds than the normal individuals who were not predisposed to hallucinate and the non-hallucinating psychiatric patients. In addition, they noted that the normal individuals who were predisposed to hallucinate were significantly more likely to see suggested objects than their respective controls, although this finding was not replicated in the psychiatric subjects. These results indicate that strong suggestions are more likely to induce hallucinatory experiences in predisposed normal individuals and in psychiatric patients with underlying hallucinatory tendencies.

HALLUCINATIONS IN DISSOCIATIVE STATES

Like hypnosis, dissociative states involve alterations of consciousness that may be induced by suggestion or may occur spontaneously. In such states there is a lack of reality testing and a lack of sense of reality that lead to depersonalization, derealization, hallucinatory phenomena, and temporary personality disorganization.

Bourguignon (1970) studied numerous societies with regard to their cultural and ritualistic behavior that involved altered states of consciousness such as dissociative states, fugue states, hypnotic states and states of "possession trance" and "simple trance." She made clear distinction between "possession trance" and "trance." According to Bourguignon (1970), in "possession trance," the individual may believe that spirits have invaded his or her body and may then perform accordingly in a ritualistic manner. While in "trance," the individual experiences various visions of a hallucinatory nature which may be private, and do not lead to behavioral changes.

As in hypnosis, hallucinatory symptoms in dissociative states represent breakthroughs of unconscious material into consciousness for the purpose of wish fulfillment, expression of repressed impulses, or other psychodynamic conflicts. The hallucination of a feared object serves to defend the individual against anxiety stemming from the conflict by distancing the self from the source of the conflict (Kessler, 1972); i.e., experiencing the source of the anxiety as external. Rothstein (1981) argued that dissociative hallucinations represent a state of regression to an earlier stage of ego functioning during which thoughts are equivalent to actual images.

Kessler (1972) suggested that dissociative reactions occur more frequently in adolescents who may be particularly vulnerable to such phenomena due to increased sexual desires, high suggestibility, emotional lability, and striving for mastery of identity issues. Further discussion involving hallucinations in dissociative states is provided in Chapter 6.

HYSTERICAL PSYCHOSIS

This condition is analogous to hysterical somatic symptoms in the sense that it represents an unconscious conflict that seeks expression through a psychological route. Furthermore, hysterical psychotic reactions may help the individual to avoid an activity or to get support from the environment. This condition is also known as "pseudopsychosis," and it involves the occurrence of sudden episodes of hallucinations and delusions without thought disorder, mood changes, or other psychiatric findings (Bishop & Holt, 1980).

Goodwin et al. (1971) reported that hallucinatory symptoms of several modalities have been observed in patients diagnosed to have "hysteria" based on their chronic multiple somatic complaints in the absence of a known medical disease. Most of those patients were aware of the unreality of their experiences.

McKegney (1967, 1987) suggested that some patients experience hallucinations as conversion symptoms. He proposed that such perceptions may represent a revival of experiences that occurred in the past at the time of satisfying relationships. He noted that most of these hallucinations occurred under psychological stress. It was later argued by Asaad and Shapiro (1987) that these experiences as reported by McKegney may, in fact, represent pseudohallucinations that arise during altered states of consciousness or dissociative states as indicated earlier.

HYPNAGOGIC AND HYPNOPOMPIC HALLUCINATIONS

The term "hypnagogic" is derived from the Greek words "hypnos" which means "sleep" and "agogos" which means "leading." "Hypnopompic" is also derived from the Greek words "hypnos" and "pompe," the latter word meaning "going away" (Weiner, 1961). Consequently, hypnagogic hallucinations refer to hallucinatory symptoms that occur during the period preceding falling asleep, whereas hypnopompic hallucinations occur during the transition from sleep into wakefulness. It is obvious that these hallucinations occur during states of altered consciousness and are closely related to sleep physiology. As mentioned earlier (Chapter 4), these hallucinations fall between dreams and true hallucinations. Furthermore, it has been suggested that hypnagogic hallucinations may become incorporated into dreams, and that dreams can turn into hypnopompic hallucinations (Savage, 1975).

Hypnagogic and hypnopompic hallucinations occur frequently in normal people, and they are mostly of the visual modality, however, auditory hallucinations may also occur. These hallucinations may be experienced with great clarity and intensity.

In addition, kinesthetic hypnagogic hallucinations are common. An example of such an experience is when the sleeper sees a ball thrown toward her. The sleeper immediately will respond with a jerking reflex to catch the ball. Another example is when a person dreams of missing a step or stumbling, a kinesthetic hallucination may occur in which the individual senses the loss of balance, followed immediately by a jerking reflex recovery movement that may be strong enough to awaken him (West, 1975).

At times paraesthesia or the sense of paralysis in the mouth and the extremities may occur. In such instances, the person dreams that he or she is in a dangerous situation. In the dream, the person may then attempt to escape or scream for help, but not be able to produce any sound, or move his or her legs. These hallucinations are described as transient dream-like experiences that are rarely confused with reality. It has been suggested that these hallucinatory experiences do not reflect any underlying psychopathology, rather, they seem to be related to the person's capacity to produce mental imagery. In any event, the content of such hallucinations generally reflects the underlying emotional state and is usually influenced by environmental factors (Vihvelin, 1948).

Hypnagogic and hypnopompic hallucinations occur particularly in children and adolescents, and in individuals who are under physical or emotional stress. They are also found frequently in individuals with psychotic disorders and as part of the clinical manifestations of narcolepsy syndrome (McDonald, 1971).

Hypnagogic hallucinations are considered primary symptoms of narcolepsy. They occur in association with sleep paralysis during the transition from waking to REM sleep, within minutes after falling asleep. The hallucinations are of a dream-like nature and consist of auditory and visual perceptions, usually with a terrifying quality (Wittig et al., 1983). The individual is usually aware of the unreality of the perceptions. Episodes of irresistible sleep may occur following meals or during monotonous situations. Other symptoms include loss of muscle tone (cataplexy) that may occur following emotional events such as laughing (Simonds, 1986).

Although it is believed that hypnagogic and hypnopompic hallucinations are related to sleep physiological phenomena and dreams, the exact mechanism of their production is still unknown. West (1975) hypothesized that as the individual falls asleep, he or she passes rapidly through a zone in which awareness of the environment is decreased, but the level of cortical arousal is still high. This discrepancy between cortical arousal and decreased environmental awareness may lead to hypnagogic hallucinations. Similarly, as the person is waking up, the same zone is passed through in which cortical arousal increases but awareness of the environment has not yet taken place. This, in turn, leads to the occurrence of hypnopompic hallucinations.

A particular form of hypnagogic hallucinations, known as the "Isakower phenomenon," consists of vague visual images of large objects perceived as approaching the face of the individual and receding away from it. This phenomenon may occur while falling asleep or upon awakening. The individual may experience a gritty sensation around the mouth, which may be associated with a milky, salty taste. Isakower phenomenon is believed, in psychoanalytic thinking, to represent a reawakening of the memory of early nursing experiences (Isakower, 1938). However, Cavenar and Caudill (1979) offered further explanations. They suggested that this phenomenon may reflect anxiety that results from oral frustration and may serve as a regressive defense, or it may simply be associated with dreams.

SUMMARY

Hallucinatory symptoms can be induced in some individuals under hypnosis or during dissociative states. Within this context, hallucinations serve the function of facilitating the expression of unconscious material which then is experienced by the individual as existing in the external world. Hypnagogic and hypnopompic hallucinations represent related phenomena that usually occur under normal conditions.

15

Hallucinations in Nonmorbid Conditions

Hallucinatory phenomena have long been known to occur in normal healthy individuals under certain conditions. Though the incidence of these experiences in the normal population is not documented, Stevenson (1983) suggested that many members of the general population, at one time or another, have experienced one or several memorable hallucinatory perceptions. He reported that several surveys in Great Britain and the United States have shown that between 10 percent and 27 percent of the general population has reported some type of hallucinatory experience, often in the visual modality, that involves the sensory perception of the presence of another person, when, in fact, no one was physically present.

Although these vague hallucinatory perceptions may occur under normal circumstances, more elaborate and definite hallucinations can occur in some people who are subjected to abnormal environmental conditions, such as prolonged sensory deprivation, sleep deprivation, starvation, and severe stress.

HALLUCINATIONS SECONDARY TO SENSORY DEPRIVATION

West (1962, 1975) considered sensory deprivation an essential factor in the mechanism responsible for hallucinatory phenomena. He hypothesized that the decrease or absence of external stimulation allows certain perceptions or "traces" that had been stored earlier in the brain to emerge into consciousness and be experienced as hallucinations.

Several experiments have been conducted to assess the effect of sensory deprivation on mental functions. Hallucinatory experiences of all sensory modalities have been produced under such conditions. Other psychiatric symptoms such as anxiety, depression, disorientation, withdrawal, and sleep disturbances have also been reported (Kellerman et al., 1977).

Zuckerman and Cohen (1964) reviewed the results of 40 sensory deprivation studies. They reported that both visual as well as auditory hallucinations

100

occurred in the subjects. Some people experienced unformed "meaningless" sensations such as flashes of light, spots, and simple geometric patterns, whereas others reported true "meaningful" hallucinatory experiences consisting of integrated scenes. The authors noted that many of the studies showed that hallucinatory perceptions progressed gradually from simple "meaningless" sensations into integrated "meaningful" true hallucinations as sensory deprivation continued over time.

As was discussed earlier (Chapter 12), visual hallucinations occur in various forms of eye disease that lead to partial or complete blindness due to deprivation of visual sensory input. Similarly, auditory hallucinations may also follow partial or complete deafness resulting from various types of ear disease that decrease or eliminate auditory sensory input for a prolonged period.

HALLUCINATIONS SECONDARY TO SLEEP DEPRIVATION AND SLEEP CYCLE DISTURBANCES

Some writers and researchers have indicated that lack of sleep may precipitate hallucinatory experiences in certain individuals. Baldwin (1970) reviewed the reports of several authors and noted that hallucinations occurred in subjects following waking periods of at least 72 hours and were particularly marked after 96 hours of sleep deprivation. He added that EEG recordings of these subjects showed a decline in alpha activity. (As discussed in Chapter 4, Itil (1970) has found a correlation between certain hallucinatory experiences and decreased alpha activity). Most hallucinations consisted of visual experiences of flashing lights or spectral color. However, auditory hallucinations in the form of noises were reported occasionally. A few subjects experienced dream-like visions of a complex nature on rare occasions.

Mullaney et al. (1983) studied 30 volunteer college students during sustained continuous performance that lasted for 42 hours. He noted that visual hallucinations, visual illusions, depersonalization, and disorientation occurred more frequently in those subjects who performed consistently without a nap or a break. Such experiences decreased in frequency as subjects were allowed to take one hour naps on regular intervals. No hallucinatory phenomena were reported in subjects who were allowed a six hour sleep in the middle of the 42 hour experiment. The results reported by Mullaney et al. (1983) suggest that a combination of sleep deprivation and fatigue, sustained concentration and effort, restriction of sensory input and circadian effects may have contributed to the hallucinatory experiences.

Snyder (1983) reported the occurrence of isolated sleep paralysis as well as transitory auditory and visual hallucinations in individuals on prolonged flights that involved rapid time zone changes ("jet lag"). He suggested that these experiences might have been caused by relative sleep deprivation, changes in REM sleep, and fluctuations in circadian rhythms. The relationship between hallucinations and sleep was discussed in greater detail in Chapter 4.

HALLUCINATIONS SECONDARY TO SEVERE FOOD AND WATER DEPRIVATION

It has been suggested that severe food and water deprivation may set the stage for hallucinations. Such experiences have been reported during general starvation as has occurred in prisoner of war camps (Baldwin, 1970). Forrer (1960) reviewed various circumstances that led to "benign" auditory and visual hallucinations and indicated that the occurrence of hallucinatory experiences following severe hunger and thirst suggests that hallucinatory phenomena may be viewed ultimately as a process with a physiological origin. Conn (1947) reported that hallucinatory symptoms could occur during hypoglycemic states in the absence of seizure activity.

HALLUCINATIONS ASSOCIATED WITH SEVERE FATIGUE

It has been shown by Mullaney et al. (1983) that severe fatigue caused by sustained continuous performance was, among other factors, involved in the production of visual hallucinations, depersonalization, and disorientation among college students who participated in their study. They indicated that as the subjects continued to work without rest, the ability to perform the assigned tasks deteriorated rapidly, and the psychological disturbances began to appear.

HALLUCINATIONS INDUCED BY LIFE-THREATENING STRESS

People who are subjected to life-threatening situations, such as rape, being taken hostage, or near death accidents may later develop visual, auditory, or tactile hallucinations in the form of recurrent intrusive experiences for a long time after the original stressful event had taken place. Siegel (1984) studied victims of rape, kidnapping, and terrorism. The individuals had a history of being subjected to various conditions of isolation, visual deprivation, restraint of physical movement, physical abuse, and threat of death. The author reported that eight subjects out of the total 31 individuals who participated in the study experienced visual hallucinations that progressed from simple geometric images to complex memory images of the traumatic event coupled with dissociative states. He noted that hallucinations occurred only in those subjects who had been subjected to both isolation and life-threatening stress.

As was discussed earlier (Chapter 6), people with post-traumatic stress disorder may experience recurrent hallucinatory perceptions of various modalities in the form of "flashbacks" in addition to feelings of anxiety, agitation, depersonalization, derealization, and other psychological and behavioral disturbances.

HALLUCINATIONS EXPERIENCED BY POST-RESUSCITATION PATIENTS

It is reported by some individuals who have been resuscitated following "clinical death" that they had experienced perceptions in which they saw certain scenes and images and heard sounds and conversations. These individuals reported having had these experiences during both "dying" and revival. The experience is described as a dream-like state sometimes accompanied by depersonalization. Though it has been suggested that these perceptions may represent manifestations of an after-life phenomena, Negovsky (1984) argued that such auditory and visual perceptions are the product of physiological changes that occur during "dying" and the reversal of the process that occurs during resuscitation. Therefore, it is questionable whether these perceptions are in fact hallucinatory in nature, or whether they simply represent pathophysiological activity within the brain that is caused by "clinical death" and revival.

HALLUCINATIONS ASSOCIATED WITH GRIEF REACTION

During grief periods, some people may experience hallucinations, such as seeing or hearing the deceased. Usually the person is quite aware of the unreality of the perceptions. It is generally believed that such experiences reflect the underlying psychodynamic wish to reexperience being with the deceased during the grief period. Shen (1986) reported a case of a 24-year-old, half Hopi Pueblo Indian male who, following the death of his father, developed a prolonged course of hallucinatory symptoms concerning the deceased. The author suggested that hallucinatory experiences facilitate the release of intensive feelings. However, he pointed out that such prolonged hallucinations may occur specifically among the Hopi Indians during the mourning process.

Frantz (1984) indicated that some of the symptoms that can accompany normal grief reactions may include depression and paranoia in addition to hallucinations of seeing the dead person. Wells (1983) stated that pathologic grief reactions may precipitate hallucinatory symptoms that are not related to seeing or hearing the deceased. He described two such cases in which the individuals reported visual hallucinations of the self or a substitute. He suggested that such experiences may be related to autoscopic phenomena (see Chapter 2).

PHANTOM LIMB SYNDROME

It has long been noted that persons who lose a limb may continue to experience various perceptions arising from the amputated limb. Such experiences include feelings of pain or movement in the limb. These kinaesthetic hallucinations may also occur in paralyzed limbs (Lishman, 1987).

Weiner (1961) indicated that sensations arising from the amputated limb tend to diminish when sensory input from the stump is increased either by massage of the stump or by use of a prosthesis. This suggests that perceptions arising from the amputated extremity may be related to sensory deprivation.

Phantom breast sensations have also been reported. Jarvis (1970) conducted an investigation among women who underwent mastectomy. He found that 23 percent of the women studied had experienced phantom breast sensations such as itching or pain. These sensations were described as having started two to six months after the surgery. Although he acknowledged that these phenomena may bear little clinical significance, Jarvis (1970) noted that such sensations were more common among younger women, especially if the surgery was performed before the menopause. He added that the sensations were more likely to be reported by women who had experienced post-operative edema in the arm. Furthermore, phantom sensations occurred more frequently in women who suffered from post-mastectomy depression.

HALLUCINATED PAIN

Hallucinations of touch (tactile hallucinations) may take various forms, such as feelings of paraesthesia, vibration, or pain. In the absence of an organic or psychiatric condition that may contribute to the hallucinatory experience, hallucinations of pain may be understood in the context of hysterical reaction or suggestion.

Forrer (1970) noted that hallucinated pain may be differentiated from actual pain by the fact that the former is vague, uncertain, and does not follow neuroanatomical boundaries in its distribution. In addition, hallucinated pain seems to occur under certain psychological circumstances and may be ameliorated by specific activities.

HALLUCINATIONS AND CULTURAL INFLUENCES

Hallucinatory symptoms have been experienced by people from many regions and diverse cultures. The social significance of such phenomena has varied from one culture to another. Certain ancient cultures regarded hallucinatory experiences acquired by eating certain mushrooms as "motif for war," "hereditary pleasures," or "divine ecstasy" (Baldwin, 1970). On the other hand, other cultures with fundamentalist religious beliefs viewed hallucinatory experiences, induced under strong suggestions or in dissociative states, as means to express the conflict between good and evil (Simonds, 1986). In some cultures, the belief in evil spirits, ghosts, or other supernatural creatures may be reinforced by the ability of certain individuals within the culture to experience visual hallucinations that involve repeated citings of such entities (Leon, 1975).

Kroll and Bachrach (1982) compared the religious hallucinations of 23 psychiatric patients with descriptions of visions from the Middle Ages. The authors noted that there were many points of similarity between the two classes of phenomena and pointed out that none of the medieval visionaries had been identified as mentally ill. They suggested that cultural norms have a central role in determining the attribution of mental illness.

HALLUCINATIONS IN EXCEPTIONAL PEOPLE

Related to the cultural influences, is the notion that some exceptional people throughout history have been described to have "special powers" that enabled them to see or hear things that others did not. It is believed that hallucinations have occurred among individuals such as Socrates, Joan of Arc, Mohammad, Luther, Pascal, William Blake, Bunyan, Napoleon, Raphael, and Goethe (Medlicott, 1958). These hallucinations, in the absence of a morbid etiology, may be viewed as caused by forms of strong suggestions, dissociative states, or prolonged sensory deprivation.

HALLUCINATIONS AND CREATIVE THOUGHT

It has been suggested by some authors that hallucinations may be seen as experiences on a continuum of the thinking process. Bauer (1970) argued that there is a similarity between sequences of thought process during problem solving and the experience of hallucination. He elaborated that during a hallucinatory experience a person may go through certain essential phases such as "preparation," "incubation," and "illumination," all of which have been attributed to creative thinkers. He added that the experience of hallucinations is very similar to the moment of "illumination" in an "act of discovery." The views presented by Bauer are not supported by clinical or research evidence.

HYPNOSIS, SUGGESTION, AND TRANCE STATES

Hallucinatory symptoms have been described to occur in the course of dissociative states, strong suggestions, or hysteria. These phenomena are considered nonmorbid experiences, even though they tend to occur more frequently in certain susceptible individuals and in certain cultures. Details of such hallucinations are offered in Chapter 14.

HALLUCINATIONS OR PSEUDOHALLUCINATIONS

It is clear that, in most instances of hallucinatory experiences occurring in nonmorbid conditions, the individual is usually quite aware of the unreality of the experience. Furthermore, such hallucinations tend to be brief, transient, and are usually influenced by certain environmental factors. It may be more accurate to refer to these perceptions as "pseudohallucinations." On the other hand, Stevenson (1983) proposed the term "ideophany," which means "private appearance," to describe all unshared sensory experiences that occur in nonmorbid conditions. This term has not been adopted by writers in the psychiatric field.

SUMMARY

Various forms of hallucinatory phenomena are reported to occur in normal healthy individuals under certain conditions, for example, sensory deprivation, sleep deprivation, starvation, severe fatigue, life-threatening stress, grief reactions, and cultural influences. Most of these hallucinations may be referred to as pseudohallucinations.

16

Hallucinations: Diagnostic Considerations

Hallucinations occur in a wide variety of psychiatric and nonpsychiatric conditions, and they represent major psychiatric symptoms that require special attention and careful examination. The clinical presentation of hallucinatory symptoms may vary considerably from one condition to another, and from one patient to another, even among those who suffer from the same disorder. The clinical characteristics of hallucinations are heavily influenced by biological, environmental, and psychodynamic factors.

Hallucinations may present in one or more of several sensory modalities; they can be auditory, visual, tactile, olfactory, or gustatory. They can vary in complexity from simple unformed perceptions to formed and elaborate experiences. They may be persistent and intense or transient and mild. They can be accompanied by other psychiatric symptoms, such as delusions and thought disorder, or by physical symptoms and behavioral disturbances. Some patients are aware of the unreality of the experiences, whereas others firmly believe in their existence. Most of time, the content of the hallucination reflects the underlying psychodynamic theme of the individual's condition. Careful assessment of the clinical characteristics of hallucinatory symptoms may provide the clinician with useful insight that can help in establishing an accurate diagnosis and, consequently, in rendering the appropriate treatment.

DIAGNOSTIC SIGNIFICANCE OF HALLUCINATIONS

Hallucinations are often referred to in clinical practice as target symptoms—used to evaluate the patient's improvement or deterioration. Questioning patients about the presence or absence of these symptoms is an essential part of mental status examination. Positive reporting of such experiences usually alerts the clinician to the possible existence of significant psychopathology that requires further investigation and evaluation.

Although they can be easily identified and monitored, hallucinations seem to have a limited diagnostic value due to their lack of specificity. It is important to emphasize that any particular type of hallucinations may be encountered in several different psychiatric and medical conditions. Furthermore, any specific disorder may manifest with different types of hallucinations in different patients. Additionally, patients who have hallucinations involving one sensory modality at one time may experience hallucinations involving other modalities at other times (Asaad & Shapiro, 1986).

Goodwin et al. (1971) conducted a study to evaluate the diagnostic significance of hallucinations in several psychiatric conditions. The sample included 117 psychiatric inpatients who carried the diagnoses of schizophrenia, affective disorders, alcoholism, organic brain syndromes, or hysteria. The authors found that hallucinatory symptoms were nonspecific and did not seem to offer adequate diagnostic value. Auditory hallucinations were reported in schizophrenia, affective disorders, and alcoholism almost with equal frequency. Visual hallucinations were also common in all diagnostic groups. Tactile and olfactory hallucinations were reported more frequently in hysterical patients. Goodwin et al. (1971) also found that most patients reported experiencing hallucinatory perceptions that involved more than one sensory modality.

Other researchers have noted the diversity of hallucinatory symptoms among schizophrenic patients. Small et al. (1966) studied 50 schizophrenics with regard to their hallucinatory symptoms. They found that auditory hallucinations occurred in 66 percent, visual hallucinations in 30 percent, tactile hallucinations in 42 percent, and olfactory hallucinations in 38 percent of all patients. Bowman and Raymond (1931) noted that visual hallucinations occurred in 22 percent of schizophrenics and in 17 percent of manic depressive patients.

Hellerstein et al. (1987) looked at the clinical significance of auditory hallucinations among psychiatric patients. They compared 151 patients who reported auditory hallucinations with 638 patients who did not report such symptoms. The authors noted that the presence of auditory hallucinations was significantly associated with the diagnosis of schizophrenia. In addition, they found that patients with hallucinations were significantly younger, had significantly fewer brief hospitalizations, and required more frequent use of maximal observation, physical restraints, and seclusion as compared with the nonhallucinating patients.

Looking specifically at the clinical significance of command hallucinations, Hellerstein et al. (1987) compared hallucinating patients who reported command hallucinations (N=58) with those who experienced non-command auditory hallucinations (N=93). The authors found that the two groups were not significantly different on demographic and behavioral variables, such as suicidal and assaultive behavior, or regarding the need to use maximal observation, seclusion, and physical restraints. They concluded that command hallucinations alone may not imply greater risks of acute life-threatening behavior.

These findings should be viewed with caution as such patients are generally very disturbed and still require special attention and observation.

The fact that hallucinations have a limited diagnostic specificity should not discourage the clinician from exploring these symptoms in all patients for two important reasons. First, hallucinations may still provide the clinician with useful diagnostic information when assessed in conjunction with other signs and symptoms, and, hence, they may support and enhance the diagnostic impression. Second, although they are generally nonspecific, hallucinations in certain disorders tend to have particular common features that manifest more frequently in those disorders as compared with others. This may help the clinician pursue specific leads in one direction or another during the clinical evaluation, based on the characteristics of the hallucinatory symptoms.

ORGANIC VERSUS "FUNCTIONAL" MENTAL DISORDERS

Although it has been argued that hallucinations are not diagnostic of any specific condition, there are several common features that characterize hallucinatory symptoms as they occur in various disorders. For example, hallucinations in organic mental disorders are mainly visual, with mostly simple and unformed perceptions. Auditory hallucinations occur less frequently in such states and are also unformed. Other types of hallucinations can occur depending on the nature of the organicity. In these conditions, the individual is often aware of the unreality of the experiences.

On the other hand, hallucinations in "functional" psychiatric conditions are mainly auditory, although other modalities may be involved as well. In any event, the hallucinatory experience usually consists of complex and elaborate perceptions, and seems to be consistent with other psychotic symptoms that may be present, i.e., patients who believe that people are out to kill them may hallucinate threats being made against them. These patients are usually convinced that these perceptions are actually originating from the external world.

As it has been emphasized, these characteristics represent clinical impressions that are based on the frequency of occurrence of particular hallucinatory symptoms in certain conditions, and are by no means diagnostic of one disorder or another. It is well known, for example, that schizophrenic patients may experience visual hallucinations of simple unformed nature. Similarly, patients with alcohol hallucinosis can experience auditory hallucinations of a complex and even commanding nature that are very difficult to differentiate from schizophrenic hallucinations. The general guidelines presented above are useful only if applied cautiously and if considered within the context of the whole history and the clinical presentation of the disorder.

"Functional" psychiatric disorders generally refer to conditions that do not have a clearly defined organic etiology. However, current thinking and research evidence suggest that most psychiatric disorders commonly referred to as "functional" do, in fact, have an underlying organic etiology, the exact nature of which is not yet fully understood. The recent explosion in the field of neuropsychiatry and molecular neurobiology is providing many clues in this regard. Cummings (1988) has suggested the use of the term "idiopathic" instead of "functional" to refer to such conditions as schizophrenia, affective disorders, and other psychiatric diseases of poorly understood etiology.

DIFFERENTIAL DIAGNOSIS

Hallucinations of schizophrenia are often in the auditory modality, and involve complex and elaborate content that is consistent with the general theme of the psychiatric state. Frequently the patient reports two voices talking about him or her in the third person. In addition, command hallucinations are typical of schizophrenia, although they occur in alcohol hallucinosis as well. Simple unformed hallucinations may occur in schizophrenia, and certain schizophrenic patients may present mainly with visual hallucinations as their major symptoms. Additionally, tactile, olfactory, and gustatory hallucinations can occur in some schizophrenics (Goodwin et al., 1971).

Auditory hallucinations may be perceived as coming from outside of the head or from within the head. This difference does not seem to imply a significant diagnostic value. However, it is believed that patients who perceive the voices as coming from inside the head may have a less severely distorted sense of reality, and they may be closer to those "healthier" patients who report that the voices they hear represent their own thoughts.

Gruber et al. (1984) investigated the laterality of auditory hallucinations in 29 psychiatric patients with various psychiatric disorders. They found that patients with right-sided hallucinations showed significantly higher scores on the Hamilton rating scale of depression as compared with those patients with left-sided or unlocalized hallucinations. Patients who experienced right-sided voices reported exclusively negative content of their hallucinations. The authors suggested that these findings may have some implications for the function of each hemisphere concerning the processing of affect and the relationship between psychotic and affective pathology. Tanabe et al. (1986), after reporting a case of right-sided complex auditory hallucinations following a hemorrhagic infarction in the left superior temporal gyrus, concluded that the lateralization phenomena of complex auditory hallucinations may provide some significant clinical sign indicating the presence of an injury in the superior temporal gyrus opposite to the hallucination side (see Chapter 11).

Hallucinations that occur in bipolar disorders, psychotic depression, schizophreniform disorders, and other "functional" psychiatric conditions may resemble to a great extent those encountered in schizophrenia. A careful examination of the longitudinal course of the illness, the level of functioning, and the presence or absence of other psychiatric symptoms is essential in making a useful and accurate differential diagnosis.

As discussed earlier, hallucinations in organic mental disorders are usually visual and unformed. However, other sensory modalities can be involved, and complex hallucinations can occur as well. Here too, careful history and examination are necessary in order to investigate any possible organic factor that may contribute to the clinical presentation. Physical examination and laboratory tests are indispensable in cases of suspected organic etiology.

Within various types of organic mental disorders, the differential diagnosis may be extremely difficult. It is even more difficult to correlate certain hallucinatory symptoms with specific causes or localized regions within the brain. It has been suggested, for example, that unformed visual hallucinations of an ictal nature are associated with occipital lobe lesions, whereas formed visual hallucinations may occur in temporal lobe injury. On the other hand, "release" visual hallucinations are usually formed and complex regardless of the location of the lesion (Cummings & Miller, 1987). Chapter 11 elaborates on this subject.

Hallucinations associated with alcoholism may be very difficult to differentiate from those seen in other psychiatric conditions (Goodwin et al., 1971). Hallucinations that occur during delirium tremens are usually visual or tactile, whereas those of alcohol hallucinosis are often auditory and may resemble greatly schizophrenic hallucinations. Furthermore, alcohol hallucinosis may be commanding in nature and may drive the patient into dangerous behavior. It is especially difficult to differentiate hallucinations resulting from a primary psychiatric disorder from those arising from substance abuse in patients who carry both diagnoses (see Chapter 7).

The clinical characteristics of various hallucinatory symptoms as they occur in different psychiatric and organic conditions are further discussed in various chapters throughout this book.

CLINICAL CONSIDERATIONS

In attempting to make a differential diagnosis utilizing hallucinatory symptoms as a guideline, the clinician needs to pay attention to several factors. It is important to identify the sensory modality of hallucinations and the degree of complexity of the experience. The content of the hallucination should be evaluated in light of the general theme of the psychiatric illness. It is also important to assess the degree to which the experience is being perceived as real or as unreal, and to consider the degree of its vividness. In addition, it is essential to evaluate the pattern, the frequency, and the duration of the hallucination, and the associated features such as certain ideas, emotions or feelings that trigger or accompany the experience. Finally, it is extremely important to assess the patient's degree of insight and how much the hallucinations affect his or her judgment, and the extent to which he or she is likely to act as a consequence of the hallucinatory experience (West, 1975).

SUMMARY

Hallucinatory symptoms seem to have a limited diagnostic value due to the relative lack of specificity in their type, complexity, and content, as they present in various disorders. However, when assessed in conjunction with other psychiatric and medical symptoms, they can enhance the diagnostic impression, and help the clinician understand the underlying psychodynamic issues.

17 =

Treatment of Hallucinations

Hallucinatory symptoms are relatively easy to identify and monitor, and are often referred to by clinicians to evaluate the patient's improvement or deterioration. Hallucinations that occur in the course of a psychotic condition are treated, along with other psychotic symptoms, with neuroleptics and other therapeutic interventions. In some instances hallucinations may disappear in response to proper treatment while other psychotic symptoms such as paranoid delusions persist. In other instances, most of the psychotic symptoms may improve significantly leaving the patient with residual hallucinatory symptoms. Clinical variability in responsiveness of hallucinations to treatment is largely determined by the underlying etiology of the disorder. Treatment of hallucinations that occur due to an organic condition should be directed at the underlying causative disturbance, although other treatments such as the administration of an antipsychotic medication may be essential until the organic condition is resolved. In addition, there are certain clinical conditions that manifest solely with hallucinatory symptoms, such as alcohol hallucinosis, which become the only target for the treatment.

PHARMACOLOGIC TREATMENT

Antipsychotic Medications

To date, antipsychotic medications remain the most specific and effective drugs for the treatment of psychotic symptoms, including hallucinations. The dosage needed and the duration of the treatment varies from one condition to another. Treatment of hallucinatory symptoms resulting from organic psychotic states, as in the case of delirium or drug-induced psychosis, may be accomplished by using a relatively small dose of a high potency neuroleptic for few days or weeks at most. On the other hand, in attempting to treat hallucinations in the course of a chronic psychotic condition, such as schizophrenia, the physician may need to prescribe much larger amounts of the medication and for a longer duration. There is no clinical evidence that a certain antipsychotic drug may be superior to another in its efficacy in controlling hallucinatory symptoms. The drug is best chosen based on the patient's past history of responding to that medication and on the side effect profile of the drug in relation to the clinical condition. The patient should be placed on the appropriate dose and for an adequate length of time before the medication is declared ineffective. In most cases changing from one neuroleptic to another may offer little advantage, however, some patients may show better response to one drug than they do to others.

Lithium Preparations

Lithium is well known for its antimanic as well as its antidepressant effects. It has been suggested in the past few years that lithium may exert some antipsychotic effects as well. Zemlan et al. (1984) investigated the effect of lithium therapy on core psychotic symptoms of schizophrenia and schizoaffective disorder. They reported that psychotic symptoms, including hallucinations, delusions, and thought disorder responded favorably to lithium therapy in a relatively short period of time. They concluded that lithium could be regarded as a more rapidly acting antipsychotic agent than it is normally assumed. Lithium may be used in some hallucinating patients who fail to respond to traditional neuroleptic treatment.

Carbamazepine

The anticonvulsant carbamazepine, commercially known as Tegretol, has received increasing attention in the past few years concerning its applications in psychiatric disorders. The drug is widely used at present as an effective agent for the treatment of bipolar disorders. It is also used to improve poor impulse control in some patients with certain personality disorders or organic mental conditions that manifest with behavioral disturbances. There have been a few recent reports that identified carbamazepine as an effective drug for the treatment of hallucinations. Kraft et al. (1984) reported the case of a woman who had a sudden onset of auditory hallucinations associated with depressive symptoms that lasted for three years. The patient did not respond to antidepressants, antipsychotic medications, or to ECT. Her EEG did not show any gross abnormalities. The patient was started on 600 mg. of carbamazepine per day, and in three days her hallucinations decreased markedly, however, her depressive symptoms did not change.

Neppe (1988a), on the other hand, doubted the conclusions drawn by Kraft et al. (1984) and reported the case of a man with a complex partial seizure disorder with no past history of hallucinations or any psychotic symptoms who developed auditory "pseudohallucinations" as a result of rapid reduction in his carbamazepine dosage from 1400 mg./day to 400 mg./day. The voices disappeared after the dosage was increased to the previous level. Neppe (1988a) hypothesized that the hallucinatory symptoms were due to withdrawal from carbamazepine.

Wells (1985) suggested that patients with persistent organic hallucinosis resulting from prolonged use of heavy hallucinogenic drugs in the past may respond favorably to anticonvulsant medications.

Benzodiazepines

The role of benzodiazepines in the treatment of psychoses continues to be a controversial one among clinicians. It is generally agreed upon that benzodiazepines may be used in combination with antipsychotic medications in the treatment of acute psychotic states in order to reduce the level of the patient's agitation. Furthermore, benzodiazepines are used with good results in cases of acute psychotic reactions induced by psychedelic drugs. Additionally, benzodiazepines are considered the specific treatment of choice in cases of delirium tremens resulting from alcohol or benzodiazepine withdrawal, in which visual and tactile hallucinations are very common.

It has been argued recently that benzodiazepines may have a specific effect on psychotic symptoms including hallucinations. Lingiaerde (1982) reported on the effect of the benzodiazepine derivative estazolam on a group of chronic schizophrenics who experienced auditory and visual hallucinations among other symptoms. The patients who participated in the study had failed to respond to neuroleptics alone. After a few weeks of treatment with estazolam in addition to the neuroleptics, the patients showed significant improvement in their hallucinations and in their general clinical condition. Lewis (1985) reported that he had been able to relieve chronic intractable hallucinosis in nine of 12 patients who suffered from residual schizophrenia by using benzodiazepines. He described one patient with chronic auditory hallucinations in addition to other psychotic symptoms who improved dramatically after he was started on oxazepam 5 mg. tid. The hallucinosis recurred when the patient stopped taking the oxazepam. Jos et al. (1985) reported the cases of two patients whose hallucinations responded to treatment with diazepam. The first patient had refractory hallucinations that persisted despite an ECT course which helped with her depressive and other psychotic symptoms. After failing to respond to several psychotropic agents over the course of four years, the patient was started on diazepam 5 mg. tid, which led to complete suppression of the hallucinations within one day. The recovery lasted for four months after which time the hallucinations recurred despite the continuation of the same treatment, however, the patient was not significantly distressed by her hallucinations. The second patient, a chronic schizophrenic with a history of head injury and seizure disorder, who had suffered from psychotic symptoms that included visual and auditory hallucinations, failed to respond to antipsychotics or to anticonvulsant medications. A regimen of 40 mg. of diazepam per day resulted in a significant decrease in his anxiety and hallucinations within days. When the dose was increased to 60 mg. per day, the visual hallucinations were totally eliminated and the auditory hallucinations were greatly suppressed. It is worth noting that both patients were being maintained on antipsychotic medications in addition to diazepam throughout the course of the treatment. Greenberg et al. (1986) reported the case of a patient who developed psychotic symptoms following modest oral use of "what was probably" an amphetamine in addition to smoking marijuana. The symptoms consisted of auditory hallucinations, delusions, and thought broadcasting, and they persisted despite his prompt stopping the use of these substances. In addition, depressive symptoms were noted. The patient was treated with lorazepam 1 mg. per day with prompt relief of his psychotic symptoms including the auditory hallucinations.

Other Pharmacologic Treatments

Khantzian (1983) reported an extreme case of cocaine dependence that was complicated with paranoid delusions, auditory, visual and tactile hallucinations, and suicidal feelings. The patient was given methylphenidate 15 mg. tid. Within 24 hours, there was rapid resolution of all delusion and hallucinations and other acute symptoms. The author suggested that methylphenidate might be useful in treating cocaine dependence and might alleviate craving behavior, as well as toxic and withdrawal symptoms that might include hallucinations.

ENVIRONMENTAL MODIFICATIONS

Several approaches that involve manipulation of environmental stimulation and the patient's perception have been attempted in order to alleviate hallucinations with variable degrees of success.

It has been suggested that increasing external auditory stimulation may decrease the likelihood of auditory hallucinations. Margo et al. (1981) investigated the effect of variations of auditory input on hallucinatory experiences in schizophrenic patients. Their results suggest that stimulation in itself is not enough to reduce the hallucinatory experience in a significant way, but rather, the structure present in the material used for stimulation and its ability to command the patient's attention are what may determine the effect on hallucinatory phenomena. Feder (1982), referring to the same principle, reported the case of a 29-year-old patient with chronic auditory hallucinations who was successfully treated by listening to a radio through stereo headphones. Magen (1983) reported the case of a schizophrenic patient who stated that her auditory and visual hallucinations increased after her television set had broken. She noted that watching television had markedly decreased both her auditory and visual hallucinations.

Manipulation of auditory input by wearing an earplug on one side was reported by some authors to decrease auditory hallucinations. Done et al. (1986) succeeded in reducing persistent auditory hallucinations in a patient by utilizing this technique. They noted that beneficial effects of wearing an earplug were detected only when the plug was inserted in the dominant ear. Prior to this, James (1983) reported somewhat different findings. He treated two schizophrenic patients who had persistent auditory hallucinations and who had failed to respond to neuroleptic medications. Both patients were treated by inserting an earplug which was moved from side to side during the treatment. Both patients showed significant improvement whether the earplug was on the dominant or the non-dominant side. However, the improvement rate slowed after transferring the earplug from one side to the other.

BEHAVIORAL MODIFICATIONS

As was suggested earlier, auditory hallucinations in some schizophrenic patients may be accompanied by subvocal speech. Bick and Kinsbourne (1987) noted that 14 of 18 hallucinating schizophrenic patients reported that the voices they heard went away when they undertook a maneuver that consisted essentially of opening the mouth wide. The maneuver seemed to abolish subvocalizations along with hallucinations. Evenson (1987) reported that similar results could be achieved by asking patients to hum a tune when they wanted the voices to stop. He added that this method requires some practice in order to become effective. It is important to add here that similar techniques that involve using the vocal apparatus to alleviate auditory hallucinations were reported over 20 years ago by Erickson and Gustafson (1968) who asked their patients to gargle, hum, sing, or simply talk in order to ameliorate their auditory hallucinations.

Fonagy and Slade (1982) applied aversive conditioning techniques to treat auditory hallucinations of chronic schizophrenics. They reported that the most successful outcome occurred when white noise was presented concurrently with hallucinatory reports made by patients.

Alford et al. (1982) suggested that a cognitive approach may be effective in alleviating hallucinatory symptoms. They reported that verbal therapy sessions that addressed the hallucinatory-delusional behavior resulted in a temporary but marked decrease in the behavior. Johnson et al. (1983) reported the case of a 30-year-old patient who suffered from recurrent visual hallucinations and obsessional ruminations. The patient was treated with thought-stopping techniques that resulted in improvement in his obsessional thoughts and produced marked decrease in the frequency of the hallucinations. Later the patient was treated with an anger-induction technique that resulted in complete remission of his hallucinations. Lamontagne et al. (1983) assessed the effect of thought-stopping on delusions and hallucinations in chronic schizophrenic patients. They concluded that using this technique in addition to antipsychotic medications produced significantly better results than did using antipsychotics alone.

Falloon and Talbot (1981) explored various strategies used by 40 chronic schizophrenic outpatients to cope with their persistent auditory hallucinations. They noted that several coping mechanisms were utilized with good results, including changes in activity, interpersonal contact, manipulations of physiological arousal, and attentional control.

PSYCHOTHERAPY

It must be emphasized here that psychotheraputic interventions need to be implemented in addition to any other treatment modality used in the management of hallucinations. The type of psychotherapy may vary depending on the nature of the illness and on the individual patient. Patients who develop hallucinations as part of an organic mental disorder may or may not be aware of the unreality of their perceptions. In all events, it becomes essential to reassure patients and to explain to them the nature of their experiences, and the fact that the symptoms will probably disappear with proper treatment. On the other hand, schizophrenic patients and others with "functional" psychotic conditions may be convinced that their hallucinations are real. Here too it is important to support the patients and to educate them about their illness. It should be acknowledged that the perceptions they are reporting are actually experienced by them, and are not a product of their imagination, yet they are caused by the illness. The degree of insight that can be reached about the hallucinations will depend on the degree of improvement of patients' sense of reality and on their cognitive and intellectual level.

Taylor (1983) illustrated the feasibility of applying psychoanalytic principles on hallucinatory symptoms in certain patients. He described the analysis of a psychotic female graduate student who presented with delusions and chronic auditory hallucinations as well as a wide variety of visual hallucinations. Taylor (1983) applied certain aspects of Melanie Klein's work focusing on the patient's communications and object relationships as they related to her hallucinatory symptomatology, which resulted in significant improvement.

On the other extreme, patients with simple and concrete thinking may respond well to a more supportive approach. For example, Neppe (1988b) reported the case of a 34-year-old patient with auditory hallucinations, probably secondary to complex partial seizures, who decided to tape record the voices that he was hearing. The patient was rather astonished to discover that the voices did not appear on the tape. This experience prompted the patient to see his physician because he realized that he must be ill. Neppe (1988b) suggested that tape recording auditory hallucinations by patients may have an indirect therapeutic application for non-schizophrenic hallucinating patients such as those with underlying organic disorders. He felt that this technique might allow patients to gain some insight into the unreality of their perceptions and, hence, help them cope with their unpleasant experiences.

Finally, there are those patients whose hallucinations are ego-syntonic and are often pleasant and enjoyable. Such patients may look forward to the occurrence of their hallucinations, and learn to adapt quietly to them. In most of these cases, the nature and the content of the hallucinations seem to fulfill certain wishes or unconscious needs that may help the patient adapt to the external world. In such instances, therapeutic interventions may not be necessary.

OTHER TREATMENT MODALITIES

The efficacy of electroconvulsive therapy (ECT) in certain psychiatric disorders has been widely documented in the literature. One of the major indications for ECT is major depression with psychotic features in which hallucinations and delusions may be present. The response to ECT in those instances is usually quite favorable. This procedure is particularly useful and safe in elderly patients who have medical complications, especially those who cannot tolerate psychotropic medications. ECT may also be given in cases of extreme mania in which psychotic symptoms may or may not be present. The efficacy of ECT in the treatment of schizophrenia is somewhat controversial and is probably less favorable than in affective disorders. However, some patients who have failed to respond to antipsychotic medications may do well following a course of ECT (Taylor & Fleminger, 1980).

There had been some reports in the literature that suggested that schizophrenic symptoms have decreased after hemodialysis therapy (Wagemaker & Cade, 1977). However, such conclusions were later challenged by several investigators who were unable to produce the same results, and, therefore, did not support the contention of the therapeutic efficacy of hemodialysis in schizophrenia (Carpenter, 1987).

Finally, it may be of interest to the reader to mention the potential benefits of "psychosurgery" in cases of intractable hallucinations. Although "psychosurgery" remains highly controversial and still limited to extreme intractable psychiatric conditions due to ethical, moral, and legal reasons, some patients with severe and persistent hallucinations who have failed to respond to any other treatment modality may benefit from such a procedure. Maurizi (1985) suggested that hallucinatory symptoms may respond well to bilateral resection of the superior sympathetic ganglion, or to elimination of the sympathetic nerve supply to the pineal gland.

18 =

Toward an Integrative Theory of Hallucinations

We have observed that hallucinatory phenomena can occur in a wide variety of disorders and situations that may be seen as lying along a spectrum. On one side of the spectrum, we see normal people who may experience hallucinations under certain circumstances such as sensory deprivation, hypnotic states, grief, or under the influence of certain drugs. On the other side of the spectrum, we see severely disturbed patients with chronic psychotic conditions such as schizophrenia or manic depressive disorder. Along the spectrum, we come across patients with various psychiatric and organic conditions that may present with variable degrees and forms of hallucinatory symptoms.

Any attempt to integrate current knowledge, as it relates to the mechanism of hallucinations, into a comprehensive model must begin with the assumption that there have to be some universal aspects that exist in all hallucinatory states. It has been suggested repeatedly, in the past as well as in recent years, that dreams represent a hallucinatory state that occurs during sleep. Hallucinations during sleep do occur regularly in otherwise healthy individuals as part of the normal psychological/physiological process of dreaming (Asaad & Shapiro, 1986). In addition, certain people, who are otherwise healthy individuals, can be made to hallucinate under certain circumstances that may alter specific physiological or biochemical mechanisms within the brain, such as the administration of a variety of drugs, or the exposure to certain abnormal conditions, such as severe exhaustion, sleep deprivation, or sensory deprivation. Other people who have psychiatric or organic disorders seem to hallucinate as the result of a pathological process that involves the Central Nervous System.

Therefore, it appears that all people experience hallucinatory phenomena in one form or another, during waking state or in dreams. How do we account for a phenomenon that, on the one hand, is distinctly abnormal when it occurs in the course of certain psychiatric or organic illness during the waking state that constitutes two-thirds of our lives, yet on the other

120

hand, is clearly part of normal functioning when it occurs in the one-third of life in which we sleep?

In order to answer this question, any integrative theory of hallucinations must postulate the failure of a central screening mechanism that controls the flow of stimuli from both the external environment and the brain, and serves the function of excluding extraneous stimuli that are not relevant to attentiveness. This mechanism is normally in operation during waking states and non-REM sleep and is "turned off" during REM sleep. The mechanism may also be "turned off" during waking states in the presence of certain pathological processes, toxic states, or abnormal physiological conditions (West, 1962, 1975). Furthermore, it is likely that the "on-off switch" is mediated through a group of several neurotransmitters that are influenced by physiological as well as pathological changes.

It has long been postulated that the most likely site for such a mechanism is the brain stem. Scheibel and Scheibel (1962) suggested that although hallucinations are mostly generated within the brain stem, they are not exclusive products of that site. They added that such phenomena may also be produced by experimental or pathologic manipulations of the various structures within the central nervous system, from the brain stem to ultimate cortical levels. However they emphasized that the brain-stem reticular core may play a central role in hallucinatory phenomena, since it is the only system that appears to be involved anatomically and physiologically at each or at all of the levels from the brain stem to the cortex.

Several writers have reported on the association between brain stem pathology and hallucinatory phenomena. Roberts et al. (1983) demonstrated that intrinsic brain-stem pathology may be responsible for psychotic symptoms including hallucinations. Cascino and Adams (1986) suggested that auditory hallucinations are caused by lesions of the tegmentum of the pons and lower mid-brain. Lindstrom et al. (1987) concluded in a recent experiment that brain stem dysfunction is involved in the psychopathology of auditory hallucinations in schizophrenic patients, probably by interfering with the auditory pathways in the brain stem. Additionally, evidence from normal dream physiology, sleep EEG studies, and nonpsychiatric disease states such as narcolepsy (REM-type) points toward the brain stem as the major anatomical site for the "on-off/screening mechanism" that may be responsible for controlling hallucinatory phenomena.

The correlation between hallucinations and REM sleep has been documented repeatedly throughout the literature. This relationship can be explained in light of the brain stem being the anatomic site for the "on-off/screening mechanism." Several researchers have suggested that hallucinations of delirium tremens and other deliria, arising from withdrawal from substances that suppress REM sleep, are produced by the intrusion of dreams of REM sleep into wakefulness during the rebound phase (Greenberg & Pearlman, 1967). Hypnagogic and hypnopompic hallucinations and hallucinatory symptoms encountered in cases of narcolepsy may be explained by a similar mechanism (Roth, 1980). Furthermore, it has been proposed that hallucinations of schizophrenia and mania may be produced by the intrusion of certain components of REM sleep into the wake period (Maurizi, 1985).

In any event, it seems that a defective screening mechanism which may be mediated through the reticular formation system at the brain-stem level may allow hallucinatory phenomena to occur in all conditions discussed above. The screening mechanism may become defective under certain physiological or pathological situations in which specific neurotransmitters play an essential role. Hallucinogenic drugs and all other pharmacologic agents that are known to induce hallucinatory symptoms are likely to produce "toxic" effects that may disrupt the normal flow of neurotransmitters throughout the central nervous system, including the brain stem where the "on-off/screening mechanism" becomes dysfunctional allowing hallucinatory experiences to occur.

Ictal hallucinations and hallucinatory symptoms produced as a result of brain injuries, tumors, infections, and similar conditions may represent a somewhat different and probably a distinct variety of hallucinations. It has been shown that spontaneous or iatrogenic stimulation of the occipital cortex may lead to simple unformed visual hallucinations, yet stimulation of the temporal cortex often produces formed hallucinatory images (Cummings & Miller, 1987). However, it is likely that even these forms of hallucinations are regulated by a brain-stem mechanism; that is, a descending aminergic or other neurotransmitter tracts may relay the impulses from the peripheral cortical areas into centers within the brain stem and, hence, influence brain-stem biochemistry leading to hallucinatory phenomena.

In the "functionally" psychotic patient, it is likely that there is a neurotransmitter-mediated or CNS-receptor-mediated dysfunction that permits failure of the normal operation of the screening mechanism and, thus, the emergence of hallucinatory symptoms. It is most likely that the vulnerability to hallucinate is largely dictated by the tendency of that "on-off/screening mechanism" to become dysfunctional under certain physiological or pathological conditions. According to current research, the biological basis of hallucinatory vulnerability is most likely linked to pathological processes in post-synaptic catecholamine, indolamine, and cholinergic receptor site and/or a neuro-regulatory imbalance among a number of normally interacting neurotransmitter chemical systems. In schizophrenia, other "functional" psychotic states, and organic mental disorders, these systems become largely dysfunctional due to imbalances or abnormal interactions among various neurotransmitters. However, in general, and in the absence of a major psychiatric or organic condition, these systems are likely to be mostly "fluid" and liable to be influenced by several environmental variables, such as sensory deprivation, sleep-wake cycle disruption, chemical intoxication, or, perhaps, psychologically induced "stressors."

It is likely that pathological neurochemistry or receptor neurophysiology represents the neural substrate for the psychoanalytic concept of "weak ego." Clinical variations in individual ego strengths may reflect underlying variable degrees of biological vulnerability. The "match-mismatch" model proposed by Klein et al. (1980), which emphasizes that the person's ability to test reality is dependent on the ability of the CNS to match external stimuli to previously stored experiences, is probably another way of expressing the same view. Here one might also add that the ability of the CNS to perform this function may well be regulated by healthy neurotransmission.

Another important and unresolved area is whether early life experiences may induce or create a greater vulnerability to psychosis or to hallucinations. For such a hypothesis to be likely, an environmental stressor or simply an environmental change must lead to physiological and biochemical changes within the CNS, and, consequently, alter the vulnerability of the individual to future environmental or endogenous stressors. The work of Kandel and Schwartz (1981), which indicates that the actual structure of CNS synapses may be altered by environmental changes, is in line with this type of thinking. This kind of research might point toward how early exposure to certain environmental factors may influence actual CNS structure and, thereby, have a pathogenic influence (Asaad & Shapiro, 1986).

The content of hallucinations in almost all conditions is clearly related to previous life experience and unconscious material. In this sense, hallucinations appear to serve a function similar to that served by dreams, and the two phenomena become most alike. In both situations, repressed unconscious wishes or impulses are projected as voices or images coming from the outside world. Psychodynamic concepts of hallucinations seem to complement biological theories and offer another dimension to the phenomena that involves human emotions and behavior.

It is important to keep in mind that hallucinations occur in a broadly heterogeneous population. Thus, for some individuals, these expressions of biological vulnerability are likely to occur under almost any circumstance, whereas for others, there must be a specific interplay between a certain biological vulnerability and a specific environmental stressor.

Although the "on-off/screening mechanism" theory within the brain stem is a very likely hypothesis that can account for most hallucinatory states, hallucinations remain a very complex phenomenon, and are still far from being fully understood or explained by any single mechanism. It is clear, however, that hallucinations are produced as a result of an interplay among several physiological, biochemical, and psychodynamic variables, and they may well represent a final common pathway that involves biological vulnerability and psychological influences (Asaad & Shapiro, 1986).

Hallucinations have been described in a wide variety of clinical conditions and disorders ranging from non-morbid conditions, to purely organic disorders, to vaguely understood "functional" psychotic states. They have been prominent hallmarks of mental illness throughout recorded history, and continue to be major psychiatric symptoms to the present day. It is likely that further exploration of these leading symptoms of psychosis may provide us with a better understanding of the underlying etiology and pathogenesis of schizophrenia and other psychiatric disorders in general. Freud stated that dreams are the royal road to the unconscious. It may very well be that further research involving the mechanisms of hallucinations will lead the way to uncovering the mysteries of mental illness.

References

Adair, D.K., & Keshavan, M.S. (1988). The Charles Bonnet Syndrome and grief reaction. (letter) *American Journal of Psychiatry, 145* (7), 895–896.

Aizenberg, D., Schwartz, B., & Modai, I. (1986). Musical hallucinations, acquired deafness, and depression. *The Journal of Nervous and Mental Disease, 174* (5), 309–311.

Albala, A.A., Weinberg, N., & Allen, S.M. (1983). Maprotiline-induced hypnopompic hallucinations. *Journal of Clinical Psychiatry, 44* (4), 149–150.

Alexander, L. (1970). Hypnotically induced hallucinations: Their diagnostic and therapeutic utilization. In W. Keup (Ed.), *Origin and Mechanisms of Hallucinations.* New York: Plenum Press.

Alford, G.S., Fleece, L., & Rothblum, E. (1982): Hallucinatory-delusional verbalizations: Modification in a chronic schizophrenic by self-control and cognitive restructuring. *Behavior Modification, 6* (3), 421–435.

Allen, J.R. (1985). Salicylate-induced musical perceptions (letter). *The New England Journal of Medicine, 313* (10), 642–643.

Allen, T., & Agus, B. (1968). Hyperventilation leading to hallucinations. *American Journal of Psychiatry, 125,* 632–637.

Altshuler, K.Z. (1971). Studies of the deaf: Relevance to psychiatric theory. *American Journal of Psychiatry, 127,* 1521–1526.

Ambrosetto, G. (1986). Post-ictal gustatory hallucinations, sleep related microspikes and glioma of the Sylvian region: Report of a case. *Clinical Electroencephalography, 17* (2), 89–91.

Arieti, S. (1974). *Interpretation of Schizophrenia,* 2nd ed. New York: Basic Books.

Aristotle, De Somnis (1941). In R. McKeon (Ed.), *The basic works of Aristotle.* New York: Random House.

Asaad, G., & Shapiro, B. (1986). Hallucinations: Theoretical and clinical overview. *American Journal of Psychiatry, 143,* 1088–1097.

Asaad, G., & Shapiro, B. (1987). Hallucinations as conversion symptoms (Reply Letter). *American Journal of Psychiatry, 144,* 696–697.

Asaad, G. (1988). Atypical presentations of manic depressive disorder. *Resident and Staff Physician, 34,*(4) 73–75.

Asaad, G. (1989). Relationship between illusions, hallucinations, and delusions. *Integrative Psychiatry, 6,* 196–198.

Askenasy, J.J., Gruskiewicz, J., Braun, J., & Hackett, P. (1986). Repetitive visual images in severe war head injuries. *Resuscitation, 13,*(3) 191–201.

Bachman, D.M. (1984). Formed visual hallucinations after metrizamide myelography. *American Journal of Ophthalmology, 97,* 78–81.

Baldwin, M. (1970). Neurologic syndromes and hallucinations. In W. Keup (Ed.), *Origin and Mechanisms of Hallucinations.* New York: Plenum Press.

Ballenger, J.C., & Post, R. M. (1978). Kindling as a model for alcoholic withdrawal syndrome. *British Journal of Psychiatry, 133,* 1–14.

.X. (1970). Hypnosis, suggestions, and auditory-visual "hallucinations": A
ical analysis. In W. Keup (Ed.), *Origin and Mechanisms of Hallucinations.*
New York: Plenum Press.

es, F.F. (1982). Precipitation of mania and visual hallucinations by amoxapine
hydrochloride. *Comprehensive Psychiatry, 23* (6), 590–592.

Bartlett, J.E.A. (1951). A case of organized visual hallucinations in an old man with
cataract, and their relation to the phenomena of the phantom limb. *Brain, 74.*
363–373.

Bauer, S.F. (1970). The function of hallucinations: An inquiry into the relationship of
hallucinatory experience to creative thought. In W. Keup (Ed.), *Origin and
Mechanisms of Hallucinations.* New York: Plenum Press.

Bender, L., & Lipkowitz, H. (1940). Hallucinations in children. *American Journal of
Orthopsychiatry, 10,* 471–490.

Bender, L. (1954). Imaginary companions. In L. Bender (Ed.), *A Dynamic Psychopathology of Childhood.* Springfield, Ill.: Charles C. Thomas.

Bender, L. (1970). The maturation process and hallucinations in children. In W.
Keup (Ed.), *Origin and Mechanisms of Hallucinations.* New York: Plenum
Press.

Bennett, C.R. (1980). Nitrous oxide hallucinations (letter). *Journal of the American
Dental Association, 101* (4), 595–597.

Bentall, R.P., & Slade, P.D. (1985). Reality testing and auditory hallucinations: A
signal detection analysis. *British Journal of Clinical Psychology, 24:* 159–169.

Berrios, G.E., & Brook, P. (1982). The Charles Bonnet syndrome and the problem of
visual perceptual disorders in the elderly. *Age and Ageing, 11,* 17–23.

Bick, P.A., & Kinsbourne, M. (1987). Auditory hallucinations and subvocal speech in
schizophrenic patients. *American Journal of Psychiatry, 144,* 222–225.

Bion, W.R. (1967). *Second thoughts: Selected papers on psycho-analysis.* London:
Heinemann.

Bishop, E., & Holt, A.R. (1980). Pseudopsychosis: a reexamination of the concepts of
hysterical psychosis. *Comprehensive Psychiatry, 21,* 150–161.

Bleuler, E. (1950). *Dementia Praecox or the group of schizophrenias.* New York:
International Universities Press.

Bourguignon, E. (1970). Hallucination and trance: An anthropologist's perspective.
In W. Keup (Ed.), *Origin and Mechanisms of Hallucinations.* New York: Plenum
Press.

Bowman, K.M., & Raymond, A.F. (1931). A statistical study of hallucinations in the
manic-depressive psychoses. *American Journal of Psychiatry, 88,* 299–309.

Branchey, L., Branchey, M., Worner, T.M., Zucker, D., Shaw, S., & Lieber, C.S.
(1985). Association between amino acid alterations and hallucinations in alcoholic patients. *Biological Psychiatry, 20* (11), 1167–1173.

Brandys, Y., & Yehuda, S. (1983). Indolamine hallucinogens as MAO inhibitor agents:
A theoretical approach. *International Journal of Neuroscience, 21,* 251–256.

Brett, E.A., & Ostroff, R. (1985). Imagery and post-traumatic stress disorder: An
overview. *American Journal of Psychiatry, 142,* 417–424.

Brown, M.J., Salmon, D., & Rendell, M. (1980). Clonidine hallucinations. *Annals of
Internal Medicine, 93* (3), 456–457.

Buchsbaum, M.S., Ingvar, D.H., Kessler, R., Waters, R.N., Cappelletti, J., Van
Kammen, D.P., King, C., Johnson, J.L., & Manning, R.G. (1982). Cerebral

References

glucography with positron tomography. *Archives of General Psychia* 251–259.

Burke, P., DelBeccaro, M., McCauley, E., & Clark, C. (1985). Hallucination children. *Journal of the American Academy of Child Psychiatry, 24,* (1), 71–

Carpenter, W.T., Jr. (1987). Hemodialysis in schizophrenia (letter). *American Journa* of *Psychiatry, 144,* (6), 830.

Cascino, G.D., & Adams, R.D. (1986). Brainstem auditory hallucinosis. *Neurology, 36* (8), 1042–1047.

Cavenar, J.O., Jr., & Caudill, L.H. (1979). An Isakower phenomena variant in an initial dream. *Journal of Clinical Psychiatry, 40* (10), 437–439.

Chambers, W. (1986). Hallucinations in psychotic and depressed children. In D. Pilowsky and W. Chambers (Eds.), *Hallucinations in Children.* Washington, D.C.: American Psychiatric Press.

Chandora, D.B. (1980). Delayed diazepam withdrawal syndrome: A case of auditory and visual hallucinations and seizures. *Journal of the Medical Association of Georgia, 69* (9), 769–770.

Channer, K.S., & Stanley, S. (1983). Persistent visual hallucinations secondary to chronic solvent encephalopathy: Case report and review of the literature. *Journal of Neurology, Neurosurgery and Psychiatry, 46* (1), 83–86.

Closson, R.G. (1983). Visual hallucinations as the earliest symptom of digoxin intoxication. *Archives of Neurology, 40* (6), 386.

Cogan, D.G. (1973). Visual hallucinations as release phenomena. *Albrecht Von Graefes Archiv fur Klinische und Experimentelle Ophthalmologie, 188,* 139–150.

Cohn, R. (1971). Phantom vision. *Archives of Neurology, 25.* 468–471.

Conn, J.W. (1947). The diagnosis and management of spontaneous hypoglycemia. *The Journal of the American Medical Association, 134,* 130–137.

Cooklin, R., Sturgeon, D., & Leff, J. (1983). The relationship between auditory hallucinations and spontaneous fluctuation of skin conductance in schizophrenia. *British Journal of Psychiatry, 142,* 47–52.

Critchley, E.M., Denmark, J.C., Warren, F., & Wilson, K.A. (1981). Hallucinatory experiences of prelingually profoundly deaf schizophrenics. *British Journal of Psychiatry, 138* (1), 30–32.

Crystal, H.A., Wolfson, L.I., & Ewing, S. (1988). Visual hallucinations as first symptoms of Alzheimer's disease. *American Journal of Psychiatry, 145* (10), 1318.

Cummings, J.L., & Miller, B.L. (1987). Visual hallucinations—clinical occurrence and use in differential diagnosis. *Western Journal of Medicine, 146,* 46–51.

Cummings, J.L., Miller, B., Hill, M.A., & Neshkes, R. (1987). Neuropsychiatric aspects of multi-infarct dementia and dementia of the Alzheimer's type. *Archives of Neurology, 44,* 389–393.

Cummings, J.L. (1988). Organic psychosis. *Psychosomatics, 29* (1), 16–26.

Cunningham, B., & McKinney, P. (1983). Patient acceptance of dissociative anesthetics. *Plastic and Reconstructive Surgery, 72,* 22–26.

Damas-Mora, J., Skelton-Robinson, M., & Jenner, F.A. (1982). The Charles Bonnet syndrome in perspective. *Psychological Medicine, 12,* 251–261.

Damlouji, N.F., & Ferguson, J.M. (1984). Trazodone-induced delirium in bulimic patients. *American Journal of Psychiatry, 141* (3), 434–435.

Davis, F.A., Bergen, D., Schauf, C., McDonald, I., & Deutsch, W. (1976). Movement phosphenes in optic neuritis: A new clinical sign. *Neurology, 26,* 1100–1104.

T., & Chambers, H.E. (1978). Structure and content of hallucinations in ~ohol withdrawal and functional psychosis. *Journal of Studies on Alcohol, 39*, 1831–1840.

.ment, W., Zarcone, V., Ferguson, J., Cohen, H., Pivik, T., & Barchas, J. (1969). Some parallel findings in schizophrenic patients and serotonin-depleted cats. In D.V.S. Sankar (Ed.), *Schizophrenia: Current concepts and research*. Hicksville, N.Y.: P.J.D. Publications.

Diagnostic and Statistical Manual of Mental Disorders, Third Edition - Revised (1987). Washington, D.C.: American Psychiatric Association.

Domino, E.F., & Ruffing, M.D. (1982). Evidence for opioids as partial antagonists for indole hallucinogens. *Psychopharmacology Bulletin, 18*, 175–179.

Done, D.J., Frith, C.D., & Owens, D.C. (1986). Reducing persistent auditory hallucinations by using an ear-plug. *British Journal of Clinical Psychology, 25* (pt.2) 151–152.

Dungal, H. (1984). Visual hallucinations induced by a sympathomimetic drug. *Canadian Medical Association Journal, 131* (Nov. 15), 1186.

Dunn, D.W., Weisberg, L.A., & Nadell, J. (1983). Peduncular hallucinations caused by brainstem compression. *Neurology, 33* (10), 1960–1961.

Dunne, J.W., Leedman, P.J., & Edis, R.H. (1980). Inobvious stroke: a cause of delirium and dementia. *Australian and New Zealand Journal of Medicine, 16*, 771–778.

Dyck, P. (1985). Sylvian lipoma causing auditory hallucinations: Case report. *Neurosurgery, 16* (1), 64–67.

Egdell, H.G., & Kolven, I. (1972). Childhood hallucinations. *Journal of Child Psychology and Psychiatry and Allied Disciplines, 13*, 279–287.

Eisendrath, S.J., Matthay, M.A., Dunkel, J.A., Zimmerman, J.K., & Layzer, R.B. (1983). Guillian-Barre syndrome. Psychosocial aspects of management. *Psychosomatics, 24*, 465–475.

Ellinwood, E.H., Jr., Sudilovsky, A., & Nelson, L.M. (1973). Evolving behavior in the clinicial and experimental amphetamine (model) psychosis. *American Journal of Psychiatry, 130*, 1088–1093.

Erickson, G.D., & Gustafson, G.J. (1968). Controlling auditory hallucinations. *Hospital and Community Psychiatry, 19*, 327–329.

Esquirol, J.E.D. (1965). *Mental Maladies* (1837), New York: Hafner Press.

Evans, J.W., & Elliot, H. (1981). Screening criteria for the diagnosis of schizophrenia in deaf patients. *Archives of General Psychiatry, 38*, 787–790.

Evarts, E.V. (1962). A neurophysiologic theory of hallucinations. In L.J. West (Ed.), *Hallucinations*. New York: Grune and Stratton.

Evenson, R.C. (1987). Auditory hallucinations and subvocal speech (letter). *American Journal of Psychiatry, 144* (10), 1364–1365.

Falloon, I.R., & Talbot, R.E. (1981). Persistent auditory hallucinations: Coping mechanisms and implications for management. *Psychological Medicine, 11* (2), 329–339.

Fasullo, S., & Lupo, I. (1973). Neurophysiopathology of the visual hallucinations in delirium tremens. *Acta Neurologica, 28*, 471–480.

Feder, R. (1982). Auditory hallucinations treated by radio headphones. *American Journal of Psychiatry, 139* (9), 1188–1190.

Feinberg, I. (1962). A comparison of the visual hallucinations in schizophrenia with those induced by mescaline and LSD-25. In L.J. West (Ed.), *Hallucinations*. New York: Grune and Stratton.

Feinberg, I. (1970). Hallucinations, dreaming and REM sleep. In W. Keup (Ed.), *Origin and Mechanisms of Hallucinations*. New York: Plenum Press.

Feldman, M., & Bender, M.B. (1970). Visual illusions and hallucinations. In W. Keup (Ed.), *Origin and Mechanisms of Hallucinations*. New York: Plenum Press.

Fischer, R. (1969). The perception-hallucination continuum. *Diseases of the Nervous System, 30,* 161–171.

Fischer, R. (1970). Prediction and measurement of perceptual-behavioral change in drug-induced hallucinations. In W. Keup (Ed.), *Origin and Mechanisms of Hallucinations*. New York: Plenum Press.

Fischer, R. (1971). The flashback: Arousal state bound recall of experience. *Journal of Psychedelic Drugs, 3,* 31–39.

Fischman, L.G. (1983). Dreams, hallucinogenic drug states, and schizophrenia: A psychological and biological comparison. *Schizophrenia Bulletin, 9,* 73–94.

Fogarty, T., & Murray, G.B. (1987). Psychiatric presentation of meperidine toxicity (letter). *Journal of Clinical Psychopharmacology, 7* (2), 116–117.

Fonagy, P., & Slade, P. (1982). Punishment vs negative reinforcement in the aversive conditioning of auditory hallucinations. *Behavior Research and Therapy, 20* (5), 483–492.

Forrer, G.R. (1960). Benign auditory and visual hallucinations. *Archives of General Psychiatry, 3,* 95–98.

Forrer, G.R. (1970): The function of hallucinated pain. In W. Keup (Ed.), *Origin and Mechanisms of Hallucinations*. New York: Plenum Press.

Francis, A.F. (1979). Familial basal ganglia calcification and schizophreniform psychosis. *British Journal of Psychiatry, 135,* 360–362.

Fraser, H.S., & Carr, A.C. (1976). Propranolol psychosis. *British Journal of Psychiatry, 129,* 508–509.

Frantz, T.T. (1984). Helping parents whose child has died. *Family Therapy Collections, 8,* 11–26.

Freud, S. (1953). The interpretation of dreams (1900). In the *Complete Works of Sigmund Freud*, Standard ed., Vol. 4. London: Hogarth Press.

Frost, E. (1985). Central nervous system effects of oxide. In E. Eger (Ed.), *Nitrous Oxide/N2O*. New York: Elsevier, pp. 157–176.

Gastaut, H., & Zifkin, B.G. (1984). Ictal visual hallucinations of numerals. *Neurology, 34,* 950–953.

Gilchrist, P.N., & Kalucy, R.S. (1983): Musical hallucinations in the elderly: a variation on the theme. *Australian and New Zealand Journal of Psychiatry, 17,* 286–287.

Gillig, P., Sackellares, J.C., & Greenberg, H.S. (1988). Right hemisphere partial complex seizures: mania, hallucinations and speech disturbance during ictal events. *Epilepsia, 29* (1), 26–29.

Goetz, C.G., Tanner, C.M., & Klawans, H.L. (1982). Pharmacology of hallucinations induced by long-term drug therapy. *American Journal of Psychiatry, 139* (4), 494–497.

Goodwin, D.W., Alderson, P., & Rosenthal, R. (1971). Clinical significance of hallucinations in psychiatric disorders. *Archives of General Psychiatry, 24,* 76–80.

Green, P., & Preston, M. (1981). Reinforcement of vocal correlates of auditory hallucinations by auditory feedback: A case study. *British Journal of Psychiatry, 139:* 204–208.

Green, P. (1987). Interference between the two ears in speech comprehension and the effect of an earplug in psychiatric and cerebral-lesioned patients. In R. Takahaski, P. Flor-Henry, J. Gruzelier, & S.I. Niwa (Eds.), *Cerebral Dynamics, Laterality and Psychopathology.* Amsterdam: Elsevier.

Greenberg, R., & Pearlman, C. (1967): Delirium tremens and dreaming. *American Journal of Psychiatry, 124,* 133–142.

Greenberg, W.M., Triana, J.P., & Narajgi, B. (1986). Lorazepam in the treatment of psychotic symptoms (letter). *American Journal of Psychiatry, 143* (7), 932.

Greenblatt, D., & Shader, R. (1973). Drug therapy, anticholinergics. *New England Journal of Medicine, 288,* 1215–1219.

Grinspoon, L. (1977). *Marihuana Reconsidered* (2nd ed.). Cambridge, Mass.: Harvard University Press.

Grinspoon, L., & Bakalar, J.B. (1985). Drug dependence: Nonnarcotic agents. In H.I. Kaplan & B.J. Sadock (Eds.), *Comprehensive Textbook of Psychiatry.* Baltimore: Williams and Wilkins.

Gruber, L.N., Mangat, B.S., & Abou-Taleb, H. (1984). Laterality of auditory hallucinations in psychiatric patients. *American Journal of Psychiatry, 141* (4), 586–588.

Gunne, L.M., Lindstrom, L., & Terenius, L. (1977). Naloxone induced reversal of schizophrenic hallucinations. *Journal of Neurotransmission, 40,* 13–19.

Hachinski, V.C., Porchawka, J., & Steele, J.C. (1973). Visual symptoms in the migraine syndrome. *Neurology, 23,* 570–579.

Hall, R.C. (1983). Psychiatric effects of thyroid hormone disturbance. *Psychosomatics, 24,* 7–18.

Hammeke, T.A., McQuillen, M.P., & Cohen, B.A. (1983). Musical hallucinations associated with acquired deafness. *Journal of Neurology, Neurosurgery and Psychiatry, 46* (6), 570–572.

Hansen, C.R., Malecha M., Mackenzie, T.B., & Kroll, J. (1983). Copper and zinc deficiencies in association with depression and neurological findings. *Biological Psychiatry, 18,* 395–401.

Harris, P.L. (1984). Bromocriptine and hallucinations. *Annals of Internal Medicine, 101* (1), 149.

Harry, B., & Favazza, A.R. (1984). Brief reactive psychosis in a deaf man. *American Journal of Psychiatry, 141,* 898–899.

Hartmann, E. (1975). Dreams and other hallucinations: an approach to the underlying mechanism. In R.K. Siegel & L.J. West (Eds.), *Hallucinations: Behavior, Experience, and Theory.* New York: John Wiley & Sons.

Hausser, H.C., & Bancaud, J. (1987). Gustatory hallucinations in epileptic seizures. Electrophysiological, clinical, and anatomical correlates. *Brain, 110* (2), 339–359.

Hawks, D., Mitcheson, M., Ogborne, A., & Griffith, E. (1969). Abuse of methylamphetamines. *British Medical Journal, 2,* 715–721.

Hays, D.P., Johnson, B.F., & Perry, R. (1980). Prolonged hallucinations following a modest overdose of tripelennamine. *Clinical Toxicology, 16* (3), 331–333.

Hellerstein, D., Frosch, W., & Koenigsberg, H.W. (1987). The clinical significance of command hallucinations. *American Journal of Psychiatry, 144* (2), 219–221.

Hemmingsen, R., & Rafaelsen, O.J. (1980). Hypnagogic and hypnopompic hallucinations during amitriptyline treatment. *Acta Psychiatrica Scandinavica, 62* (4), 364–368.

Hemmingsen, R., Vorstrup, S., Clemmesen, L., Holm, S., Tfelt-Hansen, P., Sorensen, A.S., Hansen, C., Sommer, W., & Bolwig, T.G. (1988). Cerebral blood flow during delirium tremens and related clinical states studied with Xenon-133 inhalation tomography. *American Journal of Psychiatry, 145* (11), 1384–1390.

Heym, J., Rasmussen, K., & Jacobs, B. (1984). Some behavioral effects of hallucinogens are mediated by a postsynaptic serotonergic action: Evidence from single unit studies in freely moving cats. *European Journal of Pharmacology, 101,* 57–68.

Hollister, L.E. (1968). *Chemical Psychoses.* Springfield, Ill.: Charles C. Thomas.

Hooper, R., Conner, C., & Rumack, B. (1979). Acute poisoning from over-the-counter sleep preparations. *Journal of the American College of Emergency Physicians, 8,* 98–100.

Horowitz, M.J. (1969). Flashbacks: Recurrent intrusive images after the use of LSD. *American Journal of Psychiatry, 126,* 565–569.

Horowitz, M.J. & Adams, J.E. (1970). Hallucinations on brain stimulation: Evidence for revision of the Penfield hypothesis. In W. Keup (Ed.), *Origin and Mechanisms of Hallucinations.* New York: Plenum Press.

Horowitz, M.J. (1975). Hallucinations: An information-processing approach. In R.K. Siegel & L.J. West (Eds.), *Hallucinations: Behavior, Experience, and Theory.* New York: John Wiley & Sons.

Horowski, R. (1986). Psychiatric side-effects of high dose lisuride therapy in parkinsonism. *The Lancet* (August 30), 510.

Isakower, O. (1938). A contribution to the psychopathology of phenomena associated with falling asleep. *International Journal of Psychoanalysis, 19:* 331–345.

Itil, T.M. (1970). Changes in digital computer analyzed EEG during "dreams" and experimentally induced hallucinations. In W. Keup (Ed.), *Origin and Mechanisms of Hallucinations.* New York: Plenum Press.

Jackson, J.H. (1932). *Selected Writings.* London: Hoddor and Stoughton.

Jacobs, L., Feldman, M., Diamond, S.P., & Bender, M.D. (1973). Palinacousis: persistent or recurring auditory sensations. *Cortex, 9,* 275–282.

Jacobs, L., Karpik, A., Bozian, D., & Gothgen, S. (1981). Auditory-visual synesthesia. Sound-induced photisms. *Archives of Neurology, 38,* 211–216.

James, D.A. (1983). The experimental treatment of two cases of auditory hallucinations. *British Journal of Psychiatry, 143,* 515–516.

Jansson, B. (1969). The prognostic significance of various types of hallucinations in young people. *Acta Psychiatrica Scandinavica, 44,* 401–409.

Jarvik, M.E. (1970). Drugs, hallucinations and memory. In W. Keup (Ed.), *Origin and Mechanisms of Hallucinations.* New York: Plenum Press.

Jarvis, J.H. (1970). Post-mastectomy breast phantoms. In W. Keup (Ed.), *Origin and Mechanisms of Hallucinations.* New York: Plenum Press.

Jasper, H.H., & Rasmussen, T. (1958). Studies of clinical and electrical responses to deep temporal stimulation in men with some considerations of functional anatomy. *The Brain and Behavior.* Baltimore: Williams and Wilkins.

Jellema, J.G. (1987). Hallucination during sustained-release morphine and methadon administration. *The Lancet* (August 15), 392.

Johnson, C.H., Gilmore, J.D., & Shenoy, R.S. (1983). Thought-stopping and anger induction in the treatment of hallucinations and obsessional ruminations. *Psychotherapy: Theory, Research and Practice, 20* (4), 445–448.

Johnston, J.A., Lineberry, C.G., & Frieden, C.S. (1986). Prevalence of psychosis, delusions, and hallucinations in clinical trials with bupropion (letter). *American Journal of Psychiatry, 143* (9), 1192–1193.

Jones, E. (1962). *The life and work of Sigmund Freud.* New York: Basic Books.

Jos, C.J., Schneider, R., & Gannon, P. (1985). Diazepam in the treatment of hallucinations (letter). *American Journal of Psychiatry, 142* (9), 1130–1131.

Kandel, E.R., & Schwartz, J.H. (1981). *Principles of neural science.* New York: Elsevier.

Kaplan, H.I., & Sadock, B.J. (Eds.) (1985). *Comprehensive textbook of psychiatry,* 4th ed. Baltimore: Williams and Wilkins.

Keefover, R.T., Ringel, R., & Roy, E.P., 3rd. (1988). Negative hallucinations: An ictal phenomenon of partial complex seizures (letter). *Journal of Neurology, Neurosurgery and Psychiatry, 51* (3), 454–455.

Kellerman, J., Rigler, D., & Siegel, S. (1977). The psychological effects of isolation in protected environments. *American Journal of Psychiatry, 134,* 563–565.

Kerbeshian, J., & Burd, L. (1985). Auditory hallucinosis and atypical tic disorder: Case reports. *Journal of Clinical Psychiatry, 46,* 398–399.

Kessler, J. (1972). Neurosis in childhood. In B. Wolman (Ed.), *Manual of childhood psychopathology.* New York: McGraw-Hill.

Khantzian, E.J. (1983). An extreme case of cocaine dependence and marked improvement with methylphenidate treatment. *American Journal of Psychiatry, 140* (6), 784–785.

Klein, D.F., Gittelman, R., Quitkin, F., & Rifkin, A. (1980). *Diagnosis and drug treatment of psychiatric disorders: Adults and children,* 2nd edition. Baltimore: Williams and Wilkins, pp. 48–55.

Koehler, K. (1979). First rank symptoms of schizophrenia, questions concerning clinical boundaries. *British Journal of Psychiatry, 134,* 236–248.

Kolb, L.C., & Brodie, H.K.H. (1982). *Modern clinical psychiatry.* Philadelphia: W.B. Saunders.

Kornfeld, D.S., Heller, S.S., Frank, K.A., Edie, R.N., & Barsa, J. (1978). Delirium after coronary artery bypass surgery. *Journal of Thoracic and Cardiovascular Surgery, 76* (1), 93–96.

Kotsopoulos, S., Kanigsberg, J., Cote, A., & Fiedorowicz, C. (1987). Hallucinatory experiences in nonpsychotic children. *Journal of the American Academy of Child and Adolescent Psychiatry, 26* (3), 375–380.

Kraft, A.M., Hassenfeld, I.N., & Zarr, M. (1984). Response of functional hallucinations to carbamazepine (letter). *American Journal of Psychiatry, 141,* 1018.

Kroll, J., & Bachrach, B. (1982). Medieval visions and contemporary hallucinations. *Psychological Medicine, 12* (4), 709–721.

Lamontagne, Y., Audet, N., & Elie, R. (1983). Thought-stopping for delusions and hallucinations: A pilot study. *Behavioral Psychotherapy, 11* (2), 177–184.

Lanska, D.J., Lanska, M.J., & Mendez, M.F. (1987). Brainstem auditory hallucinosis. *Neurology, 37* (10), 1685.

Leon, A.C. (1975). "El duende" and other incubi: Suggestive interactions between culture, the devil and the brain. *Archives of General Psychiatry, 32,* 155–162.

Levine, A.M. (1980). Visual hallucinations and cataracts. *Ophthalmic Surgery, 11* (2), 95–98.

Lewis, M. (1982). *Clinical aspects of child development.* Philadelphia: Lee and Febiger.

Lewis, R. (1985). Relief of chronic intractable hallucinosis in residual schizophrenia with oxazepam (letter). *American Journal of Psychiatry, 142* (6), 785.

Lindstrom, L., Klockhoff, I., Svedberg, A., & Bergstrom, K. (1987). Abnormal auditory brain-stem responses in hallucinating schizophrenic patients. *British Journal of Psychiatry, 151,* 9–14.

Lingiaerde, O. (1982). Effect of the benzodiazepine derivative estazolam in patients with auditory hallucinations. A multi-centre, double-blind, cross-over study. *American Journal of Psychiatry, 139* (9), 1188–1190.

Linn, L. (1985). Clinical manifestations of psychiatric disorders. In H.I. Kaplan & B.J. Sadock (Eds.), *Comprehensive Textbook of Psychiatry,* 4th ed. Baltimore: Williams and Wilkins.

Lishman, W.A. (1987). *Organic psychiatry, the psychological consequences of cerebral disorder* (Second Edition). Oxford: Blackwell Scientific Publications.

Lloyd, E.L. (1987). Hallucinations after anaesthesia (letter). *Anaesthesia, 42* (9), 1015–1016.

Loyd, D.W., & Tsuang, M.T. (1981). A snake lady: Post-concussion syndrome manifesting visual hallucinations of snakes. *Journal of Clinical Psychiatry, 42* (6), 246–247.

Lucas, A.R., & Weiss, M. (1971). Methylphenidate hallucinosis. *The Journal of the American Medical Association, 217,* 1079–1081.

Lukianowicz, N. (1958). Autoscopic phenomena. *Archives of Neurology and Psychiatry, 80,* 199–220.

Lukianowicz, N. (1969). Hallucinations in nonpsychotic children. *Psychiatric Clinic, 2,* 321–337.

Magen, J. (1983). Increasing external stimuli to ameliorate hallucinations (letter). *American Journal of Psychiatry, 140* (2), 269–270.

Maghazaji, H. (1974). Psychiatric aspects of methylmercury poisoning. *Journal of Neurology, Neurosurgery and Psychiatry, 37,* 954–958.

Mahl, C.F., Rothenberg, A., Delgado, J.N.R., & Hamlin, H. (1964). Psychologic response in the human intracerebral electrical stimulation. *Psychosomatic Medicine, 26,* 337–368.

Malone, G.L., & Leiman, H.I. (1983). Differential diagnosis of palinacousis in a psychiatric patient. *American Journal of Psychiatry, 140* (8), 1067–1068.

Margo, A., Hemsley, D.R., & Slade, P.D. (1981). The effects of varying auditory input on schizophrenic hallucinations. *British Journal of Psychiatry, 139,* 122–127.

Marrazzi, A.S. (1970). A neuropharmacologically based concept of hallucinations and its clinical application. In W. Keup (Ed.), *Origin and Mechanisms of Hallucinations.* New York: Plenum Press.

Mathew, R.J., Duncan, G.C., Weinman, M.L. & Barr, D.L. (1982). Regional cerebral blood flow in schizophrenia. *Archives of General Psychiatry, 39,* 1121–1124.

Maurizi, C.P. (1985). The anatomy and chemistry of hallucinations and a rational surgical approach to the treatment of some schizophrenic syndromes. *Medical Hypotheses, 17,* 227–229.

Mayer-Gross, W., Slater, E., & Roth, M. (1969). *Clinical psychiatry,* 3rd. ed. London: Bailliere, Tindall and Cassell.

McDonald, G. (1971). A clinical study of hypnagogic hallucinations. *British Journal of Psychiatry, 118,* 543–547.

McKegney, F.P. (1967). Auditory hallucinations as a conversion symptom. A theoretical proposal with two case illustrations. *Comprehensive Psychiatry, 8,* 80–89.

McKegney, F.P. (1987). Hallucinations as conversion symptoms. (Letter) *American Journal of Psychiatry, 144* (5), 696.

McNamara, M.E., Heros, R.C., & Boller, F. (1982). Visual hallucinations in blindness: The Charles Bonnet syndrome. *International Journal of Neuroscience, 17* (1), 13–15.

Medlicott, R.W. (1958). An inquiry into the significance of hallucinations with special reference to their occurrence in the sane. *International Record of Medicine, 171,* 664–677.

Meltzer, H.Y., & Stahl, S.M. (1976). The dopamine hypothesis of schizophrenia: A review. *Schizophrenia Bulletin, 2,* 19–76.

Meltzer, H.Y., Arora, R.C., Jackman, H., Pscheidt, G., & Smith, M.D. (1980). Platelet monoamine oxidase and plasma amine oxidase in psychiatric patients. *Schizophrenia Bulletin, 6* (2), 213–219.

Miller, R.R. (1975). Clinical effects of pentazocine in hospitalized medical patients. *Journal of Clinical Pharmacology, 15,* 198–205.

Mills, J.A. (1974). Non-steroidal antiinflammatory drugs. Part II. *New England Journal of Medicine, 290,* 1002–1005.

Minichetti, J., & Milles, M. (1982). Hallucination and delirium reaction to intravenous diazepam administration. Case report. *Anesthesia Progress, 29* (5), 144–146.

Mintz, S., & Alpert, M. (1972). Imagery vividness, reality testing and schizophrenic hallunications. *Journal of Abnormal Psychology, 79,* 310–316.

Mize, K. (1980). Visual hallucinations following viral encephalitis: A self report. *Neuropsychologia, 18,* 193–202.

Mora, G. (1985). History of psychiatry. In H.I. Kaplan & B.J. Sadock (Eds.), *Comprehensive Textbook of Psychiatry,* 4th ed. Baltimore: Williams and Wilkins.

Moses, R.A. (1981). Entoptic and allied phenomena. In R.A. Moses (Ed.), *Adler's Physiology of the Eye. Clinical Application.* Seventh Edition. St. Louis: The C.V. Mosby Company.

Mueser, K.T., & Butler, R.W. (1987). Auditory hallucinations in combat-related chronic post-traumatic stress disorder. *American Journal of Psychiatry, 144,* 299–302.

Mulder, D., Bickford, R., & Dodge, H. (1957). Hallucinatory epilepsy: Complex hallucinations as focal seizures. *American Journal of Psychiatry, 113,* 1100–1102.

Mullaney, D.J., Kripke, D.F., Fleck, P.A., & Johnson, L.C. (1983). Sleep loss and nap effects on sustained continuous performance. *Psychophysiology, 20,* 643–651.

Nausieda, P.A., Tanner, C.M., & Klawans, H.L. (1983). Serotonergically active agents in levodopa-induced psychiatric toxicity reactions. *Advances in Neurology, 37,* 23–32.

Navia, B.A., & Price, R.W. (1986). Dementia complicating AIDS. *Psychiatric Annals, 16* (3), 158–166.

Navia, B.A., Jordan, B.D., & Price, R.W. (1986). The AIDS dementia complex, I: Clinical features. *Annals of Neurology, 19,* 517–524.

Negovsky, V.A. (1984). A neurophysiological analysis of "hallucinations" experienced by post resuscitation patients. *Resuscitation, 11,* 1–8.

Neppe, V.M. (1988a): Carbamazepine for withdrawal pseudohallucinations (letter). *American Journal of Psychiatry, 145,* 1605–1606.

Neppe, V.M. (1988b). Tape recording auditory hallucinations (letter). *American Journal of Psychiatry, 145* (10), 1316.

Nesse, R.M., Carli, T., Curtis, G.C., & Kleinman, P.D. (1983). Pseudohallucinations in cancer chemotherapy patients. *American Journal of Psychiatry, 140* (4), 483–485.

Noll, R.B., & Kulkarni, R. (1984). Complex visual hallucinations and cyclosporine. *Archives of Neurology, 41,* 329–330.

Norman, T.R., Judd, F., Holwill, B.J., & Burrows, G.D. (1982). Doxepin and visual hallucinations. *Australian and New Zealand Journal of Psychiatry, 16* (4), 295–296.

Noyes, R., Jr., Garvey, M.J., Cook, B.L., & Perry, P.J. (1988). Benzodiazepine withdrawal: A review of the evidence. *Journal of Clinical Psychiatry, 49,* 382–389.

Olbrich, H.M., Engelmeier, M.P., Pauleikhoff, D., & Waubke, T. (1987). Visual hallucinations in ophthalmology. *Graefes Archive for Clinical and Experimental Ophthalmology, 225* (3), 217–220.

Oliver, D.J. (1984). Hallucinations associated with amoxycillin? A case report. *The Practitioner, 228,* 884.

Ostow, M. (1960). The metapsychology of autoscopic phenomena. *International Journal of Psychoanalysis, 41,* 619–625.

Pakalnis, A., Drake, M.E., Jr., & Kellum, J.B. (1987). Right parieto-occipital lacunar infarction with agitation, hallucinations and delusions. *Psychosomatics, 28* (2), 95–96.

Papp, K.A., & Curtis, R.M. (1984). Cimetidine-induced psychosis in a 14-year-old girl. *Canadian Medical Association Journal, 131,* 1081–1084.

Paraskevaides, E.C. (1988). Near fatal auditory hallucinations after buprenorphine (letter). *British Medical Journal (Clinical Research Ed.), 296,* (6616), 214.

Pardal, M.M.F., Micheli, F., Asconape, J., & Paradiso, G. (1985). Neurobehavioral symptoms in caudate hemorrhage: Two cases. *Neurology, 35,* 1806–1807.

Patterson, J.F. (1988). Auditory hallucinations induced by prazosin (letter). *Journal of Clinical Psychopharmacology, 8* (3), 228.

Paulseth, J.E., & Klawans, H.L. (1985) Drug-induced behavioral disorders. In P.J. Vinken, G.W. Bruyn, H.L. Klawans (Eds.), *Handbook of Clinical Neurology,* Vol. 2. (46). Neurobehavioral disorders. Amsterdam: Elsevier.

Penfield, W., & Rasmussen, T. (1950). *The cerebral cortex of man.* New York: MacMillan.

Peroutka, S.J., Sohmer, B.H., Kumar, A.J., Folstein, M., & Robinson, R.G. (1982). Hallucinations and delusions following a right temporoparietooccipital infarction. *Johns Hopkins Medical Journal, 151* (4), 181–185.

Piaget, J. (1962). *Play dreams and imitation in childhood.* New York: W.W. Norton.

Pilowsky, D. (1986a). Problems in determining the presence of hallucinations in children. In D. Pilowsky & W. Chambers (Eds.), *Hallucinations in Children.* Washington, D.C.: American Psychiatric Press.

Pilowsky, D. (1986b): Hallucinations in children: A psychoanalytic perspective. In D. Pilowsky & W. Chambers (Eds.), *Hallucinations in Children.* Washington, D.C.: American Psychiatric Press.

Pilowsky, D., & Chambers, W. (1986). *Hallucinations in children.* Washington, D.C.: American Psychiatric Press.

Plato, Timaeus (1952). In F.M. Cornford, *Plato's Cosmology,* New York: The Humanities Press.

Portell, J. (1970). Hallucinations in pre-adolescent schizophrenic children. In W. Keup (Ed.), *Origin and Mechanisms of Hallucinations.* New York: Plenum Press.

Price, W., Coli, L., Brandstetter, R.D., & Gotz, V.P. (1985). Ranitidine associated hallucinations. *European Journal of Clinical Pharmacology, 29,* 375–376.

Price, L.H., Charney, D.S., Delgado, P.L., & Heninger, G.R. (1989). Lithium treatment and serotoninergic function. Neuroendocrine and behavioral responses to intravenous tryptophan in affective disorder. *Archives of General Psychiatry, 46,* 13–19.

Priestley, B.S., & Foree, K. (1955). Clinical significance of some entoptic phenomena. *Archives of Ophthalmology, 53,* 390–397.

Raghuram, R., Keshavan, M.D., & Channabasavanna, S.M. (1980). Musical hallucinations in a deaf, middle-aged patient. *Journal of Clinical Psychiatry, 41* (10), 357.

Rainer, J.D., Abdulah, S., & Altshuler, K.Z. (1970). Phenomenology of hallucinations in the deaf. In W. Keup (Ed.), *Origin and Mechanisms of Hallucinations.* New York: Plenum Press.

Ram, Z., Findler, G., Gutman, I., Tadmor, R., & Sahar, A. (1987). Visual hallucinations associated with pituitary adenoma. *Neurosurgery, 20* (2), 292–296.

Richardson, A., & Divyo, P. (1980). The predisposition to hallucinate. *Psychological Medicine, 10,* 715–722.

Roberts, J.K., Trimble, M.R., & Robertson, M. (1983). Schizophrenic psychosis associated with aqueduct stenosis in adults. *Journal of Neurology, Neurosurgery and Psychiatry, 46* (10), 892–898.

Robertson, C.R. (1985). Hallucinations after penicillin injection. *American Journal of Diseases of Children, 139,* 1074–1075.

Rosanski, J., & Rosen, H. (1952). Musical hallucinations in otosclerosis. *Confinia Neurologia, 12,* 49–54.

Rosenbaum, F., Harati, Y., Rolak, L., & Freedman, M. (1987). Visual hallucinations in sane people: Charles Bonnet Syndrome. *Journal of the American Geriatrics Society, 35,* 66–68.

Rosenthal, R. (1987). Visual hallucinations and suicidal ideation attributed to isosorbide dinitrate. *Psychosomatics, 28* (10), 555–556.

Roth, B. (1980). *Narcolepsy and hypersomnia.* New York: S. Karger.

Rothstein, A. (1981). Hallucinatory phenomena in children: A critique of the literature. *Journal of the American Academy of Child Psychiatry, 20,* 623–635.

Roy, C.W., & Wakefield, I.R. (1986). Baclofen pseudopsychosis: Case report. *Paraplegia, 24* (5), 318–321.

Rundell, J.R., & Murray, G.B. (1988). Visual hallucinations on low dose amitriptyline (letter). *Journal of Clinical Psychopharmacology, 8* (1), 75–76.

Safran, A.B., Kline, L.B., Glaser, J.S., & Daroff, R.B. (1981). Television-induced formed visual hallucinations and cerebral diplopia. *British Journal of Ophthalmology, 65* (10), 707–711.

Sandyk, R. (1981). Olfactory hallucinosis in Parkinson's disease (letter). *South African Medical Journal, 60* (25), 950.

Sandyk, R., & Gillman, M.A. (1985). Lithium-induced visual hallucinations: Evidence for possible opioid mediation. *Annals of Neurology, 17* (6), 619–620.

Sankey, R.J., Nunn, A.J., & Sills, J.A. (1984). Visual hallucinations in children receiving decongestants. *British Medical Journal, 288,* 1369.

Saravay, S., & Pardes, H. (1970). Auditory "elementary hallucinations" in alcohol withdrawal psychoses. In W. Keup (Ed.), *Origin and mechanisms of hallucinations.* New York: Plenum Press.

Sarbin, T.R., & Juhasz, J.B. (1975). The social context of hallucinations. In R.K. Siegel & L.J. West (Eds.), *Hallucinations: Behavior, experience, and theory.* New York: John Wiley and Sons.

Savage, C.W. (1975), The continuity of perceptual and cognitive experiences. In R.K. Siegel & L.J. West (Eds.), *Hallucinations: Behavior, experience, and theory.* New York: John Wiley and Sons.

Scheibel, M.E., & Scheibel, A.B. (1962). Hallucinations and the brain stem reticular core. In L.J. West (Ed.), *Hallucinations.* New York: Grune and Stratton.

Schreier, H.A., & Libow, J.A. (1986). Acute phobic hallucinations in very young children. *Journal of the American Academy of Child Psychiatry, 25* (4), 574–578.

Scott, D.F., Davies, D.L., & Malherbe, M.E.L. (1969). Alcoholic hallucinosis. *International Journal of the Addictions. 4,* 319–330.

Sedman, G. (1966). A comparative study of pseudo-hallucinations, imagery, and true hallucinations. *British Journal of Psychiatry, 112,* 9–17.

Segal, S.J. (1970). Imagery and reality: Can they be distinguished? In W. Keup (Ed.), *Origin and mechanisms of hallucinations.* New York: Plenum Press.

Shader, R.I. (Ed.) (1972). *Psychiatric complications of medical drugs.* New York: Raven Press.

Shapiro, B., & Spitz, H. (1976). Problems in the differential diagnosis of narcolepsy versus schizophrenia. *American Journal of Psychiatry, 133,* 1321–1323.

Shen, W.W. (1985). Potential link between hallucination and nausea/vomiting induced by alcohol? An empirical clinical finding. *Psychopathology, 18* (4), 212–217.

Shen, W.W. (1986). The Hopi Indian's mourning hallucinations. *The Journal of Nervous and Mental Disease, 174* (6), 365–367.

Siegel, R.K., & Jarvik, M.E. (1975). Drug-induced hallucinations in animals and man. In R.K. Siegel & L.J. West (Eds.), *Hallucinations: Behavior, experience and theory.* New York: John Wiley and Sons.

138   Hallucinations in Clinical Psychiatry

Siegel, R.K. (1978). Cocaine hallucinations. *American Journal of Psychiatry, 135,* 309–314.

Siegel, R.K. (1984). Hostage hallucinations: Visual imagery induced by isolation and life threatening stress. *The Journal of Nervous and Mental Disease, 172,* 264–272.

Silber, T., Chatoor, I., & White, P. (1984). Psychiatric manifestations of Systemic Lupus Erythematosus in children and adolescents. A Review. *Clinical Pediatrics, 23,* 331–335.

Silber, T., & D'Angelo, L. (1985). Psychosis and seizures following the injection of penicillin G procaine. *American Journal of Diseases of Children, 139,* 335–337.

Simonds, J. (1986). Hallucinations in children: Diagnostic considerations. In D. Pilowsky & W. Chambers (Eds.), *Hallucinations in Children.* Washington, D.C.: American Psychiatric Press.

Slade, P.D. (1976). Toward a theory of auditory hallucinations: Outline of an hypothetical four-factor model. *British Journal of Social and Clinical Psychology, 15,* 415–423.

Small, I.F., Small, J.G., & Anderson, J.M. (1966). Clinical characteristics of hallucinations of schizophrenia. *Diseases of the Nervous System, 27,* 349–353.

Snyder, S. (1983). Isolated sleep paralysis after rapid time zone change ("jet lag") syndrome. *Chronobiologia, 10,* 377–379.

Solomon, P., & Patch, V.D. (1974). *Handbook of psychiatry.* Los Altos, Calif.: Lange Medical Publications.

Stacy, C.B. (1987). Complex haptic hallucinations and palinaptia. *Cortex, 23* (2), 337–340.

Starker, S., & Jolin, A. (1982). Imagery and hallucinations in schizophrenic patients. *The Journal of Nervous and Mental Disease, 170,* 448–451.

Stearns, H.P. (1886). Auditory hallucinations in a deaf mute. *Alienist and Neurologist, 7,* 318–319.

Stevenson, I. (1983). Do we need a new word to supplement "hallucination"? *American Journal of Psychiatry, 140* (12), 1609–1611.

Strauss, J.S. (1969). Hallucinations and delusions as points on continua function. Rating scale evidence. *Archives of General Psychiatry, 21,* 581–586.

Strub, R.L., & Black, F.W. (1988). *Neurobehavioral disorders: A clinical approach.* Philadelphia: F.A. Davis Company.

Sulkava, R. (1982). Alzheimer's disease and senile dementia of the Alzheimer's type. *Acta Neurologica Scandinavica, 65,* 636–650.

Surawicz, F.G. (1980). Alcoholic hallucinosis, a missed diagnosis. Differential diagnosis and management. *Canadian Journal of Psychiatry, 25,* 57–63.

Tanabe, H., Sawada, T., Asai, H., Okuda, J., & Shiraishi, J. (1986). Lateralization phenomenon of complex auditory hallucinations. *Acta Psychiatrica Scandinavica, 74* (2), 178–182.

Taylor, D. (1983). Some observations on hallucinations: Clinical application of some developments of Melanie Klein's work. *International Journal of Psychoanalysis, 64* (3), 229–308.

Taylor, P., & Fleminger, J.J. (1980). ECT for schizophrenia. *The Lancet, 1,* 1380.

Trulson, M.E., & Jacobs, B.L. (1979a). Effects of 5-methoxy-N, N-dimethyltryptamine on behavior and raphe unit activity in freely-moving cats. *European Journal of Pharmacology, 54,* 43–50.

Trulson, M.E., & Jacobs, B.L. (1979b). Long-term amphetamine treatment decreases brain serotonin metabolism: Implementations for theories of schizophrenia. *Science, 205:* 1295–1297.

Van-den-Berg, A.A. (1986). Hallucinations after oral lorazepam in children (letter). *Anaesthesia, 41* (3), 330–331.

Van-Wieringen, A., & Vrijlandt, C.M. (1983). Ethosuximide intoxication caused by interaction with isoniazid. *Neurology, 33* (9), 1227–1228.

Vihvelin, H. (1948). On the differentiation of some typical forms of hypnagogic hallucination. *Acta Psychiatrica Scandinavica, 23,* 359.

Vike, J., Jabbari, B., & Maitland, C.G. (1984). Auditory-visual synesthesia. Report of a case with intact visual pathways. *Archives of Neurology, 41,* 680–681.

Viscott, D.S. (1968). Chlordiazepoxide and hallucinations. *Archives of General Psychiatry, 19,* 370–376.

Wagemaker, H., Jr., & Cade, R. (1977). The use of hemodialysis in chronic schizophrenia. *American Journal of Psychiatry, 134,* 684–685.

Waldfogel, S., & Mueser, K.T. (1988). Another case of chronic PTSD with auditory hallucinations (letter). *American Journal of Psychiatry, 145,* 1314.

Walker, J.I., & Cavenar, J.O., Jr. (1983). Hallucinations. In J.O. Cavenar, Jr., & K.H. Brodie (Eds.), *Signs and symptoms in psychiatry.* Philadelphia: J.B. Lippincott.

Walsh, K.P., Shelly, R.K., & Daly, P.A. (1984). Hallucinations, an unusual adverse reaction to chlorambucil. *Irish Medical Journal, 77* (9), 288–289.

Warburton, D.M., Wesnes, K., Edwards, J., & Larrad, D. (1985). Scopolamine and the sensory conditioning of hallucinations. *Neuropsychobiology, 14* (4), 198–202.

Weinberger, L.M., & Grant, F.C. (1940). Visual hallucinations and their neuro-optical correlates. *Archives of Ophthalmology, 23,* 166–199.

Weiner, M. F. (1961). Hallucinations in children. *Archives of General Psychiatry, 5,* (12), 54–63.

Wells, C.E. (1985). Organic mental disorders. In H.I. Kaplan & B.J. Sadock (Eds.), *Comprehensive textbook of psychiatry,* 4th ed. Baltimore: Williams and Wilkins.

Wells, L.A. (1983). Hallucinations associated with pathologic grief reaction. *Journal of Psychiatric Treatment and Evaluation, 5* (2–3), 259–261.

West, L.J. (1962). *Hallucinations.* New York: Grune and Stratton.

West, L.J. (1975). A Clinical and theoretical overview of hallucinatory phenomena. In R.K. Siegel & L.J. West (Eds.), *Hallucinations: Behavior, experience, and theory.* New York: John Wiley and Sons.

Westmoreland, B.E. (1980). Organic mental disorders associated with epilepsy. In H.I. Kaplan, A.M. Freedman, B.J. Sadock (Eds.), *Comprehensive Textbook of Psychiatry,* 3rd. ed., Vol. 2. Baltimore: Williams and Wilkins.

White, N.J. (1980). Complex visual hallucinations in partial blindness due to eye disease. *British Journal of Psychiatry, 136,* 284–286.

Wilcox, J.A. (1983). Psychoactive properties of benztropine and trihexyphenidyl. *Journal of Psychoactive Drugs, 15* (4), 319–321.

Wilcox, J.A. (1985). Psychoactive properties of amantadine. *Journal of Psychoactive Drugs, 17* (1), 51–53.

Wilking, V., & Paoli, C. (1966). The hallucinatory experience. *Journal of the American Academy of Child Psychiatry, 5,* 431–440.

Winters, W.D. (1975): The continuum of CNS excitatory states and hallucinations. In R.K. Siegel, L.J. West (Eds.), *Hallucinations: Behavior, experience, and theory.* New York: John Wiley & Sons.

Wittig, R., Zorick, F., Roehrs, T., Sicklesteel, J., & Roth, T. (1983). Narcolepsy in a seven-year-old child. *Journal of Pediatrics, 102,* 725–727.

Wolberg, F.L., & Ziegler, D.K. (1982). Olfactory hallucinations in migraine. *Archives of Neurology, 39* (6), 382.

Woodward, G.A., & Baldassano, R.N. (1988). Topical diphenhydramine toxicity in a five-year-old with varicella. *Pediatric Emergency Care, 4* (1), 18–20.

Wooley, D.W., & Shaw, E. (1954). A biochemical and pharmacological suggestion about certain mental disorders. *Proceedings of the National Academy of Sciences, 40,* 228–231.

Yates, D. (1980). Syncope and visual hallucinations, apparently from timolol (letter). *The Journal of the American Medical Association, 244* (8), 768–769.

Young, H.F., Bentall, R.P., Slade, P.D., & Dewey, M.E. (1987). The role of brief instructions and suggestibility in the elicitation of auditory and visual hallucinations in normal and psychiatric subjects. *The Journal of Nervous and Mental Disease, 175* (1), 41–48.

Young, J.G. (1981). Methylphenidate induced hallucinosis: Case histories and possible mechanism of action. *Journal of Developmental and Behavioral Pediatrics, 2,* 35–37.

Yudofsky, S.C., Ahern, G., & Brockman, R. (1980). Agitation, disorientation, and hallucinations in patients on cimetidine: A report of three cases and literature review. *General Hospital Psychiatry, 2* (3), 233–236.

Zemlan, F.P., Hirschowitz, J., Sautter, F.J., & Garver, D.L. (1984). Impact of lithium therapy on core psychotic symptoms of schizophrenia. *British Journal of Psychiatry, 144,* 64–69.

Zigler, E., & Levine, J. (1983). Hallucinations vs. delusions: A developmental approach. *The Journal of Nervous and Mental Disease, 171,* 141–146.

Zilboorg, G. (1935). *The medical man and the witch during the renaissance.* Baltimore: Johns Hopkins University Press.

Zuckerman, M., & Cohen, N. (1964). Sources of reports of visual and auditory sensations in perceptual-isolation experiments. *Psychological Bulletin, 62,* 1–20.

Index

Paulseth, J. E., 60, 61, 62, 63, 64, 65, 66, 91
PCP (phencyclidine), 56
Pearlman, C., *see* Greenberg, R.
Peduncular hallucinosis, 76
Pemoline, 62
Penfield, W., 22, 69
Penicillin, 67, 91
Perception, 5
Perceptual release theory, 22
Periarteritis nodosa, 77
Peroutka, S. J., 73
Personality disorders, 34
  borderline, 34
  histrionic, 35
  multiple, 36
  schizoid, 34
  schizotypal, 34
Phantom breast sensations, 104
Phantom limb syndrome, 7, 85, 104
Phantom vision, 85
Phobic disorders, 89
Phosphenes, 83
Physostigmine, 63
Piaget, J., 86
Pilowsky, D., 86, 87, 88, 92, 93
Pinel, Philippe, 2
Plato, 1, 20
Pontine-geniculate-occipital (PGO) waves, 16, 23
Porphyria, 48
Portell, J., 90
Possession, 96
Post, R. M., *see* Ballenger, J. C.
Postcardiotomy delirium, 47
Post-ictal phenomena, 71
Post-resuscitation hallucinations, 103
Post-traumatic stress disorder (PTSD), 34, 102
  in children, 89
Pot, *see* marijuana
Prelingually deaf individuals, 80
Preston, M., *see* Green, P.
Price, L. H., 62
Price, R. W., *see* Navia, B. A.
Price, W., 67
Priestly, B. S., 85
Pseudohallucinations, 7–8, 11, 12, 35, 45, 55, 60, 79, 106, 114
Pseudopsychosis, 35, 97
Psilocin, 26, 55
Psychedelic drugs, 54, 55, *see* hallucinogens

Psychodynamic theories, 18–20, 93
Psychophysiological theories, 20–24
Psychosurgery, 119

Radio headphones, 116
Rafaelsen, O. J., *see* Hemmingsen, G.
Raghuram, R., 79
Rainer, J. D., 80
Ram, Z., 73
Ranitidine, 67
Rape victims, 102
Rasmussen, T., *see* Penfield, W., *see* Jasper, H.H.
Raymond, A. F., *see* Bowman, K. M.
REM sleep, 14–17, 38, 75, 98, 121, 122
Reticular formation system, 121, 122
Retinal diseases, 82
Richardson, A., 23
Roberts, J. K., 76, 121
Robertson, C. R., 67, 91
Rosanski, J., 79
Rosen, H., *see* Rosanski, J.
Rosenbaum, F., 84
Rosenthal, R., 66
Roth, B., 122
Rothstein, A., 91, 92, 96
Roy, C. W., 67
Ruffing, M. D., *see* Domino, E. F.
Rundell, J. R., 61

Sadock, B. J., *see* Kaplan, H. I.
Safran, A. B., 74
Sandyk, R., 62, 74
Sankey, R. J., 64, 91
Saravay, S., 37
Sarbin, T. R., 4
Savage, C.W., 17, 97
Scheerer's phenomenon, 85
Scheibel, A. B., *see* Scheibel, M. E.
Scheibel, M. E., 121
Schizoaffective disorders, 33
Schizophrenia, 28–32
  in children, 90
Schizophreniform disorders, 33
Schreier, H. A., 89
Schwartz, J. H., *see* Kandel, E. R.
Scopolamine, 63
Scott, D. F., 42
Screening mechanism, 121, 122
Sedman, G., 12
Segal, S. J., 9
Sensory deprivation, 79, 81, 84, 91, 100–101, 105